OVERSIGHT HEARING ON THE FEDERAL EMPLOYEES HEALTH BENEFITS PLAN FEHBP COVERAGE OF HDC/ABMT TREATMENT FOR BREAST CANCER

HEARING

BEFORE THE

SUBCOMMITTEE ON
COMPENSATION AND EMPLOYEE BENEFITS

OF THE

COMMITTEE ON
POST OFFICE AND CIVIL SERVICE
HOUSE OF REPRESENTATIVES

ONE HUNDRED THIRD CONGRESS

SECOND SESSION

AUGUST 11, 1994

Serial No. 103–55

Printed for the use of the Committee on Post Office and Civil Service

U.S. GOVERNMENT PRINTING OFFICE

84–133   WASHINGTON : 1995

For sale by the U.S. Government Printing Office
Superintendent of Documents, Congressional Sales Office, Washington, DC 20402
ISBN 0-16-046629-6

CONTENTS

AUGUST 11, 1994

OVERSIGHT HEARING ON THE FEDERAL EMPLOYEES HEALTH BENEFITS PLAN FEHBP COVERAGE OF HDC/ABMT TREATMENT FOR BREAST CANCER

THURSDAY, AUGUST 11, 1994

House of Representatives,
Committee on Post Office and Civil Service,
Subcommittee on Compensation and Employee Benefits,
Washington, DC.

The subcommittee met, pursuant to call, at 10:00 a.m., in room 311, Cannon House Office Building, Hon. Eleanor Holmes Norton (chair of the subcommittee) presiding.

Members present: Representatives Norton, Byrne, and Morella.

Ms. NORTON. Good morning. This session will begin.

Breast cancer is probably the most dreaded of all diseases that affect women. This is to be expected of a life-threatening disease whose cure is often disfiguring. Consequently, there is necessarily strong interest whenever a new treatment proves effective. High-dose chemotherapy, or HDC, coupled with the use of autologous bone marrow transplants, or ABMT, is such a treatment. It consists of removing some bone marrow and applying extremely high doses of chemotherapy to kill the cancer. The bone marrow is then reinjected. In one study, 15 to 20 percent of patients reached a five-year cancer-free period, as compared to 1 to 2 percent treated with conventional chemotherapy.

The Office of Personnel Management has consistently refused to authorize HDC/ABMT treatment for breast cancer, although many insurance companies cover it for employees outside the Federal sector. In one case that at least raises a question concerning the possibility of sex discrimination, Blue Cross/Blue Shield covers HDC/ABMT treatment for testicular cancer, Hodgkins disease and other diseases but not breast cancer. In any case, differences in coverage for HDC/ABMT by FEHBP insurance carriers offers a compelling example of why we need health care reform. One study showed of the 533 patients studied, 412 were approved, while 121 were denied coverage by insurance carriers.

Even without an OPM mandate, some carriers cover some treatment under the auspices of the National Cancer Institute in its ongoing clinical trials.

In October 1993, I was one of 53 members of the Congress who sent a letter to OPM director, James King, requesting that he require FEHBP fee carriers to cover HDC/ABMT for cancer. Despite substantial evidence of the success for the treatment for breast cancer, OPM has taken the position that the treatment should not be used outside the clinical trial setting.

OPM's position could subject carriers to legal liabilities. Last December, an insurance carrier who refused to authorize HDC/ABMT for breast cancer treatment was ordered to pay $89.3 million to the family of a woman who subsequently had died from breast cancer. The jury believed the insurance carrier had denied coverage because of the cost of the treatment.

Is OPM's refusal to require coverage of treatment completely free of considerations of cost? There are many costly treatments for serious diseases that FEHBP insurers pay every day while remaining one of the most cost-efficient health plans in the country.

Beginning last month, Virginia now requires every health insurance company to cover HDC/ABMT treatment for breast cancer. This means the private sector employees in Virginia can get the treatment while it is denied to Federal employees in Virginia and other parts of the very same region.

Inevitably, FEHBP and the Federal government have a disproportionate effect on insurance coverage because it is one of the largest plans in the country, covering more than nine million people. Today's hearing is important, therefore, because not only will carriers within the plan treat Federal employees differently, but also because of the effect that inconsistent Federal policy surely must have on the rest of the country.

Can we afford to wait until national health care reform gets around to this issue? Can women afford to wait longer for the approval of a potentially lifesaving treatment for the leading cancer killer of women in the United States? A compelling case needs to be made if such treatment is to continue to be withheld.

We are prepared to hear both sides of the case today. Let me sincerely welcome all of today's witnesses.

May I turn now to our ranking member, Mrs. Morella, for any opening remarks she would care to make?

Mrs. MORELLA. Thank you, Madam Chairman. I appreciate you bringing the issue of the HDC/ABMT coverage for breast cancer treatment before this committee. In 1992, according to the American Cancer Society, 180,000 American women were told they had breast cancer. In that year, 46,000 women died from the disease.

When one considers that over the whole course of the war in Vietnam, 47,356 men and women sacrificed their lives as a result of combat, the enormity of those numbers is underscored by the 46,000 women who died of breast cancer in one year. Breast cancer is the most prevalent cancer among women in the United States, and it is a cancer that each year claims more and more victims. Today, it is estimated that one in eight women will be stricken. The terrible toll on women's lives and the lives of those who depend on them, their children, their spouses, their families, their friends, cannot be measured.

Current treatment methods, surgery, radiation and chemotherapy have not significantly altered mortality statistics over the past decade. We must begin to explore new promising strategies and therapies, even though there are costs and risks involved.

The issue before us today is reimbursement of high-dose chemotherapy in autologous bone marrow transplantation by insurance carriers participating in the Federal Employee Health Benefits Program. If one were to read just the testimony given on behalf of the Office of Personnel Management, one would come away with a warm feeling that the program is just about ready for complete approval. However, reading the testimony of breast cancer survivors and those who represent the medical community, one realizes that OPM and the Federal sector have been dragging their collective feet to accept ABMT as a recognized treatment for breast cancer and in directing FEHBP to reimburse for the procedure.

The question is, how long does it take for an experimental technique to become recognized as accepted procedure? How many cases must be documented? How many flip-coin cases must prove to be successful and how many years of follow-up of each case is necessary?

Madam Chair, if breast cancer patients do not get reimbursement for ABMT treatment, they are not going to submit to this extremely expensive treatment at the expense of their families, no matter how many bake sales are conducted. If patients do not submit to treatment, then there will not be enough cases to report in medical research, thereby curtailing the possibility of further developing this already proven technique.

One of the witnesses will testify that this type of treatment is—is or will be available only to the wealthy and well-educated with the tenacity to go forward with civil lawsuits against insurance companies. This is totally unacceptable. In democracy, one life is as valuable as the other, and so it should be with health care.

It is devastating for breast cancer patients to be informed by their physicians that they are ideal candidates for the ABMT treatment, only to be told by their insurance carriers that they will not be covered for the treatment. These patients often fight legal battles that take up precious time and energy. By the time they won the legal battle, they have lost the health battle because the optimum period for treatment has passed.

Madam Chair, in matters of medicine, the cautious approach is often the best path. It now appears, however, that there is sufficient medical documentation from the clinical trials and documentation projects to substantiate that high-dose chemotherapy and autologous transplantation is more effective than other conventional treatments. I have a constituent who has been through it and who points out the success and the medical bills.

I urge the Office of Personnel Management to make another evaluation and to advise participating FEHBP to include HDC/ABMT on their schedule of reimbursement coverage. I look forward to hearing the testimony by our many panels.

Thank you, Madam Chair and our distinguished colleagues.

Ms. NORTON. Thank you, Mrs. Morella.

Ms. Byrne, a Member of the subcommittee, has joined us, and I ask her if she has any opening comments.

Ms. BYRNE. Thank you, Madam Chairman.

I don't have any formal opening comments. I will just share with you and the rest the committee that not a week goes by that I don't have a phone call from either a family of a woman stricken with breast cancer or the woman herself asking for my intervention with their insurance carrier. And that by the roll of the dice in choosing an insurance carrier determines, in some cases, whether these women will actually live or die.

I think this is a very serious matter that we are taking up today and appreciate the Chair having this hearing and look forward to the testimony of those gathered.

Thank you, Madam Chair.

Ms. NORTON. Thank you, Ms. Byrne.

We are particularly pleased that the Ranking Member of the full committee has joined us, and I would ask Mr. Myers if he has any opening remarks.

Mr. MYERS. Thank you, Madam Chair. I have no prepared opening remarks. Thank you for having this hearing.

Having experienced with my wife breast cancer for the last five years, I do know something about cancer. I have an increased interest.

The other committee I serve on, Appropriations, we have come a long way. We have now mammography standards which will help the earlier diagnosis with women who will take the mammograms. But, unfortunately, in many areas of the country, mammography is not suggested or routine in women's health care. Often family doctors—I will be critical of some of them. I tell them quite frequently they should tell women that they should have mammograms. We have a witness here today who will testify to this, also. But it is a very serious problem.

And I might add that my wife had 14 months of chemo, very, very aggressive, and without surgery. It has worked. Five years ago. So we will knock on wood.

But there are treatments that are available today, but bone marrow and bone marrow harvesting is something that—and placenta, there is some research being done. I think there will be some testimony on this on the Appropriations Committee.

We are trying to advance as rapidly as science and NCI and others can work on it. We also are in the second year of a clinical test of the use of Tamoxifan. We are not sure about Tamoxifan at this point. I guess there will be some testimony on this. At least we are attempting to search in this area to find answers of, first, what causes cancer and which is the most successful treatment.

I know, as a child, I lost some friends, a friend's mother who had surgery. The only remedy back 50, 60 years ago was radical mastectomy, and it didn't work in most cases. Very seldom did it work. But we have come a long way since then. We still have a long way to go.

I thank you for this hearing. Hopefully, our granddaughters and grandsons— I might add, men have breast cancer, something that a lot of people don't understand. I know when my wife was in treatment, mostly women, of course, but it wasn't every time we were there, men were being treated, also. A little more difficult to diagnose with a man because they—mammography isn't quite as successful and men don't routinely have mammograms. But it is a disease that affects both genders. And it is and has been said, one out of nine women now sometime during their lifetime, unfortunately, with today's technology and today's experience, will experience breast cancer.

And I think, another thing, mammogram should start before the age of 50. On the health plan we are considering right now, I understand health care will only provide mammography for women after the age of 50. Well, an awful lot of great many women have breast cancer before that age.

So thank you for having this hearing. We certainly believe Federal employees are entitled to the best. Thank you.

Ms. NORTON. Thank you very much, Mr. Myers. We are pleased to have you here today.

And we are particularly pleased to welcome three Members of Congress who have very special testimony. It is an indication of the importance of this subject that these three Members would themselves come to testify. And I particularly welcome them this morning: Congresswoman Patricia Schroeder, Congresswoman Barbara Vucanovich, and Congressman Richard Lehman.

Let's start with Patricia Schroeder.

STATEMENT OF HON. PATRICIA SCHROEDER, A REPRESENTATIVE IN CONGRESS FROM THE STATE OF COLORADO

Mrs. SCHROEDER. Thank you, Madam Chair.

This is a panel that gets it. I can't tell you how honored we are to get this hearing. I think that the first time I first introduced this bill to include this in Federal employee benefits, I had no idea that maybe we would be looking at health care plans that would extend Federal employee benefits to a much broader pool. And so this hearing is even more important in dealing with this issue, is more important than we ever dreamed of when we first came across this issue.

Madam Chair, I would ask you to consent to put my statement in the record, because I note you have many more panelists, and I just want to make a few points as to how I got interested in this.

I represent a lot of Federal employees, and we came upon horror show after horror show of family members of Federal employees or Federal employees themselves coming down with breast cancer, their doctors clearly telling them bone marrow was the way to go, and then they find out that the only thing OPM could let them do is get into this clinical trial where they do a coin flip, which means half the people won't get bone marrow transplant.

Now, to have the emotional stress of a disease on people is one thing. To add to it the economic stress of can they pay for the care that is being recommended is really very tragic.

And you are going to hear from Dr. Roy Jones, who's an expert in this area, and Donna Rogers, who has been a victim of this, from Colorado, and I thank you for having them here.

Dr. Jones has shown that a five-year relapse-free survival for high-risk primary breast cancer treated with the bone marrow treatment is 35 percent better than any other result reported in the medical literature by any research group using conventional treatment. That's amazing. And yet OPM continues to insist upon having a gold standard for this that they have not required for testicular cancer or the others where they do permit payment. Why is the standard higher on breast care? Madam Chair, you put that in your opening statement, and I—I think that is a real question to ask OPM when they come up.

Secondly, in Colorado, I am a little angrier with OPM than maybe other States, because Blue Cross/Blue Shield in Colorado normally covers bone marrow transfer for—or treatment for breast cancer in the private sector, but because OPM feels they can't do it for public employees who are in the public sector, so you can imagine how happy that makes people.

We also have, obviously, the Duke University study that has looked very closely at how coverage, has looked at all of this and finds that it is really very arbitrary and capricious.

I think that we really need to get on with this. I know that I am talking to the choir. So I am going to put the rest of my statement in the record.

Thank you for moving on this and really appreciate all you are doing. Thank you.

Ms. NORTON. Thank you, Congresswoman Schroeder.

[The prepared statement of Hon. Patricia Schroeder follows:]

PREPARED STATEMENT OF HON. PATRICIA SCHROEDER, A REPRESENTATIVE IN CONGRESS FROM THE STATE OF COLORADO

Madam Chairwoman, thank you for holding today's hearing on coverage of bone marrow transplant treatment for breast cancer under the Federal Employee Health Benefits Program (FEHBP). Your commitment to federal employees is unquestionable.

I also want to thank the brave women and their families who have brought this matter to our attention. They have had to fight a terrible disease and at the same time wage a battle to pay for its treatment.

The question is whether there should be coverage beyond the National Cancer Institute's (NCI) randomized clinical trials. Let me make it clear that I support the NCI trials. But to deny women coverage under any other circumstances is, I believe, unethical.

Insurance payment should be available to patients who participate in other NCI approved treatment programs. The Office of Personnel Management (OPM) should require carriers to pay for coverage under these circumstances.

I believe there is more than enough evidence to support this policy. As Dr. Roy Jones, Director of the Bone Marrow Transplant Program at the University of Colorado, will testify, this is not a new treatment. Thousands of patients have been treated with BMT. According to Dr. Jones, the five-year relapse-free survival for high-risk primary breast cancer treated with BMT is 35 percent better than any result reported in the medical literature by any research group using any conventional treatment.

Moreover, the evidence supporting the use of bone marrow transplant treatment for breast cancer is far superior than the evidence supporting the same treatment for testicular cancer or adult neuroblastoma, both of which are not considered experimental or investigational and are not subject to general exclusion under FEHBP contracts.

There is no question a different standard has been set for determining whether bone marrow transplant treatment should be covered for breast cancer.

Finally, we will hear in other testimony how inconsistent insurance coverage is for bone marrow transplant treatment. According to a Duke University study, decisions involving coverage of bone marrow transplants for 533 patients "often seemed arbitrary and capricious."

I applaud you for holding these hearings. My own introduction to bone marrow transplant treatment came from women who were denied coverage. They were all told that their best chance to survive breast cancer was to receive bone marrow transplant treatment. They were all denied insurance coverage and most were ineligible for the clinical trials.

This hearing is for them. Thank you Madam Chair.

Ms. NORTON. Congresswoman Vucanovich.

STATEMENT OF HON. BARBARA F. VUCANOVICH, A REPRESENTATIVE IN CONGRESS FROM THE STATE OF NEVADA

Mrs. VUCANOVICH. Thank you very much, Madam Chairman, and I appreciate this opportunity to discuss the coverage of breast cancer treatments under the Federal Employee Health Benefits Program. This is a matter of importance to women and to Federal employees and to Members of Congress, and I commend you for holding this hearing.

As you may know, Madam Chairman, I was the first Member of Congress to be diagnosed with breast cancer. I had just been sworn into Congress in 1983 when I learned that I had breast cancer. At that time, the treatment choices that women have today were not available, so I did what I thought was best for me. I had a mastectomy. Had several other treatment choices been possible, my choice might have been different.

Madam Chair, I share my story with the subcommittee because things are now different than they used to be. New and promising breast cancer treatment options are available and are being tested by the National Cancer Institute. These treatment possibilities permit women with a range of options to decide what's best for them and for their families. But unless insurance companies cover such options, the choice of treatment can never be truly theirs.

Today, many health insurance plans do offer coverage for mammography and other screening measures. Insurance coverage for treatment options varies among plans, including the Federal Employee Health Benefits Program. One breast cancer treatment which is not being covered under FEHBP is high-dose chemotherapy with autologous bone marrow transplant. The National Cancer Institute is currently conducting randomized trials to determine the effectiveness of this procedure. Many in Congress believe that this procedure should be covered under FEHB.

I am not a scientist or physician, but I am a breast cancer survivor who did not have many choices at that pivotal time. I am concerned by the decision of the Office of Personnel Management to refuse to cover this service under this plan when the government's lead agency for research on cancer believes this to be a promising treatment. It almost appears that OPM has more answers about breast cancer than NCI.

Madam Chair, I believe the real question is whether FEHBP should provide reimbursement for NCI-sponsored clinical trials. Later you will hear NCI officials detail the high standards and intense scrutiny of their trial studies and investigations. Patients participating in these programs receive the best care possible, and reimbursement for this treatment should be considered. Women and men must be allowed different options for determining the course of their lives.

I appreciate the subcommittee's commitment to this issue and encourage your involvement, Madam Chair, to broaden your examination to this level. All Americans deserve more health care choices in their lives.

For the last year, Congress has examined our health care system very carefully. While Members of Congress may not agree on the changes to be made, we can all agree that the quality of health care must be maintained. NCI-sponsored trials provide the highest quality health care available to deserving patients.

I hope Congress, OPM and private insurers can work together to see that health care choice is available to patients of breast cancer and other devastating diseases. Without such treatments and without a cure for breast cancer, many lives will be lost—the lives of our mothers and our sisters and our daughters and our friends.

I applaud you and your subcommittee once again for holding this hearing on breast cancer treatments, and I hope to have the opportunity to work with you in the future.

Thank you, Madam Chair.

Ms. NORTON. Thank you. Thank you very much, Congresswoman Vucanovich.

[The prepared statement of Hon. Barbara F. Vucanovich follows:]

PREPARED STATEMENT OF HON. BARBARA F. VUCANOVICH, A REPRESENTATIVE IN CONGRESS FROM THE STATE OF NEVADA

Madam Chairman, I appreciate this opportunity to come before your Subcommittee to discuss the coverage of breast cancer treatments under the Federal Employee Health Benefit Program. This is a matter of importance to women, to federal employees and to Members of Congress and I commend you for holding this hearing.

As you know, Madam Chairman, I was the first Member of Congress to be diagnosed with breast cancer. I had just been sworn in to Congress in 1983 when I learned that I had breast cancer. At that time, the treatment choices women have today were not available so I did what I thought was best for me, I had a mastectomy. Had several other treatment choices been possible, my choice might have been different.

Madam Chairman, I share my story with the Subcommittee because things are now different than they used to be. New and promising breast cancer treatment options are now available and are being tested by the National Cancer Institute. These treatment possibilities permit women with a range of options to decide what is best for them and their families. But unless insurance companies cover such options, the choice of treatment can never truly be theirs.

Today, many health insurance plans do offer coverage for mammography and other screening measures. Insurance coverage for treatment options varies among plans, including the Federal Employee Health Benefit Program. One breast cancer treatment which is not being covered under FEHBP is high-dose chemotherapy with autologous bone marrow transplant. The National Cancer Institute is currently conducting randomized trials to determine the effectiveness of this procedure. Many in Congress believe that this procedure should be covered under FEHBP.

I am neither a scientist nor a physician, but I am a breast cancer survivor who did not have many choices at my pivotal time. I am concerned by the decision of the Office of Personnel Management to refuse to cover this service under the FEHBP, when the Government's lead agency for research on cancer believes this to be a promising treatment. It almost appears that OPM has more answers about breast cancer than NCI.

Madam Chairman, I believe the real question is whether FEHBP should provide reimbursement for NCI sponsored clinical trials. Later you will hear NCI officials detail the high standards and intense scrutiny of their trial studies and investigations. Patients participating in these programs receive the best care possible and reimbursement for this treatment should be considered. Women and men must be allowed different options for determining the course of their lives.

I appreciate the Subcommittee's commitment to this issue and encourage your involvement Madam Chairman to broaden your examination to this level. All Americans deserve more health care choices in their lives.

For the last year, Congress has examined our health care system very carefully. While Members of Congress may not agree on the changes to be made, we can all agree that the quality of health care must be maintained. NCI sponsored trials provide the highest quality health care available to deserving patients.

I hope Congress, OPM, and private insurers can work together to see that health care choice is available to patients of breast cancer and other devastating diseases. Without such treatments and without a cure for breast cancer, many lives will be lost—the lives of our mothers, our sisters, our friends.

I applaud you and your Subcommittee once again for holding this hearing on breast cancer treatments and hope to work with you in the future.

Ms. NORTON. Congressman Lehman, please.

STATEMENT OF HON. RICHARD H. LEHMAN, A REPRESENTATIVE IN CONGRESS FROM THE STATE OF CALIFORNIA

Mr. LEHMAN. Thank you very much, Madam Chair and Members of the committee. I appreciate the opportunity to testify on this issue today.

I am here today to tell you the story of Rebecca Perez-Ford, a dear family friend and former constituent of mine. She wanted to be here herself, but she is currently in the hospital undergoing treatment for her cancer. I am certain that her experience will underscore the grave need for insurance plans to cover bone marrow transplants as treatment for breast cancer.

Rebecca Perez-Ford is 39 years old, an employee of the Internal Revenue Service and currently stationed in New Orleans, Louisiana. She is the mother of three young children, ages five, three and five months. She is suffering from Stage III inflammatory breast cancer. Every oncologist involved with her case has prescribed high-dose chemotherapy with an autologous bone marrow transplant, asserting that this treatment alone offers Mrs. Ford the best hope for survival.

Miss Ford is literally fighting for her life, fighting for the opportunity to raise the young children who need her. Her struggle against cancer, however, is by no means her biggest challenge. Rather, the greatest obstacle has been a Federal insurance plan which has denied her the means to survive her disease.

Miss Ford specifically indicated to her oncologist that her insurance, Community Health Network of Louisiana, did not cover an autologous bone marrow transplant, but she was told, "Don't worry about it. It is not going to be a problem." Four days prior to her scheduled bone marrow harvest, Miss Ford was therefore shocked to receive a call from her hospital, Tulane Medical Center, advising her that her insurance would not cover the bone marrow transplant or any related procedures.

She was initially told that she would be responsible for 50 percent of the costs of the procedure. Then later she was informed that she would have to pay 100 percent of the cost. Miss Ford was then supposed to have received a number of surgical procedures and several doses of chemotherapy in preparation for the transplant. Despite the urgency of her condition, none of these were carried out as scheduled.

The hospital has since decided that they would not treat her, even on a self-pay basis. Miss Ford's pay from the IRS, where she has faithfully worked for 17 years, has run out. The donated sick leave from her co-workers has also expired.

With her chances of survival growing slimmer as each day passes, Miss Ford began looking for other ways to finance her treatment. She enlisted the aid of a lawyer to appeal the insurance company's decision. She applied for medicaid, but the time involved in processing her application would make it too late for her scheduled transplant.

As she desperately pursued the possibility of obtaining treatment from other cancer centers, she received word that a public hospital had agreed to cover the cost of the bone marrow transplant. After rescheduling at the public hospital, and thus further delaying her treatment, Miss Ford then learned that the public hospital had revoked its decision. With time running out, Miss Ford had no choice but to reschedule again. She obtained a mastectomy and could only hope that somehow she could finance a bone marrow transplant, which, in order to be effective, would have to be undertaken within approximately three weeks of the mastectomy.

It was at this point that I became aware of her unbelievable plight. Literally shocked by the endeavor she experienced, I contacted the Office of Personnel Management in the hope of expediting the appeals process. Much to my dismay, I learned that although Community Health Network had led Miss Ford to believe she could appeal her decision, OPM had no power to force the plan to cover her.

I was relieved to learn that last week Miss Ford's oncologist successfully persuaded the hospital to permit her treatment to continue. Medicaid had agreed to finance the procedure but has since also revoked its commitment, so the financial situation remains in flux.

The Federal Employees Health Benefits Program is failing miserably, Madam Chair, to address the needs of women with breast cancer. This disease, especially in advanced diagnosis, is itself a horrendous proposition. But for women like Miss Ford, everything boils down to money.

In dealing with the hospitals, the fatal illness becomes secondary as a patient's focus must be on negotiating a good price to obtain parts of a treatment plan. It is truly abhorrent that our health care system, especially the Federal Employees Federal Health Benefits Plan, leaves women to bargain for life-saving treatment.

Miss Ford exemplifies the current problem with our health care system. A diligent, middle-class woman is forced into poverty in order to receive medicaid coverage for her health care. Many FEHBP policies, including Miss Ford's, cover bone marrow transplants for testicular cancer and other diseases. OPM and the insurance companies claim that for breast cancer this procedure is not covered because it is experimental, although many noted oncologists have maintained that the evidence supporting the use of bone marrow transplants as treatment for breast cancer is far superior to the evidence supporting the same treatment for testicular cancer.

The failure of insurance plans to cover bone marrow transplants for breast cancer patients is clearly discriminatory. Insurance plans reimburse for bone marrow transplants that are far more speculative in terms of their proven speculativeness. That is unfair. It is unforgivable that women Federal employees with breast cancer are excluded from scientifically advanced medical treatment, and a revamping of OPM's policy on this issue is long overdue.

I thank the committee for hearing this testimony, and I hope you will move as quickly as you can to rectify this situation.

Ms. NORTON. Thank you very much, Congressman Lehman.

[The prepared statement of Hon. Richard H. Lehman follows:]

PREPARED STATEMENT OF HON. RICHARD H. LEHMAN, A REPRESENTATIVE IN
CONGRESS FROM THE STATE OF CALIFORNIA

I appreciate the opportunity to testify on this issue of tremendous importance to women. I am here today to tell the story of Rebecca Perez-Ford, a dear family friend and former constituent of mine—she wanted to be here herself, but she is currently in the hospital undergoing treatment for her cancer. I am certain that her experience will underscore the grave need for insurance plans to cover bone marrow transplants as treatment for breast cancer.

Rebecca Perez-Ford is thirty-nine years old, the mother of three young children, ages 5, 3, and 5 months. She is suffering from Stage III inflammatory breast cancer. Every oncologist involved with her case has prescribed high-dose chemotherapy with an autologous bone marrow transplant; they have asserted that this treatment offers Ms. Ford the best hope for survival, a 70% chance, versus 30–50% with standard treatment. Ms. Ford is literally fighting for her life, fighting for the opportunity to raise the young children who need her. Her struggle against cancer, however, is by no means her biggest challenge—rather, her greatest obstacle has been a Federal insurance plan which has denied her the means to survive her disease. By prohibiting coverage for her prescribed treatment, Community Health Network of Louisiana has left Ms. Ford defenseless against her cancer.

Ms. Ford's breast cancer was diagnosed at an advanced stage; doctors determined that her disease required an aggressive treatment plan which included chemotherapy, a mastectomy, a bone marrow transplant, and radiation—in that order. Ms. Ford specifically indicated to her oncologist that her insurance, Community Health Network of Louisiana, did not cover an autologous bone marrow transplant, but she was told "don't worry about it; it's not going to be a problem."

Four days prior to her scheduled bone marrow harvest, Ms. Ford was therefore shocked to receive a call from her hospital, Tulane Medical Center, advising her that her insurance would not cover the bone marrow transplant or any related procedures, and that she would probably be asked to pay 50% of the cost of the procedure. Two days before the scheduled commencement of her treatment, Ms. Ford was told that she would have to pay 100% of the procedure (approximately $175,000), and that in order to be admitted into the hospital, she would have to pay $4,000 and become a self-pay patient. Ms. Ford eventually received a hospital bill for $8,753 for a bone marrow harvest, instead of the $4,000 initially quoted to her.

At this point, Ms. Ford was supposed to have received a number of surgical procedures and several doses of chemotherapy in preparation for the bone marrow transplant. Despite the urgency of her condition, none of these were carried out because the insurance company could have deemed them to be related to the bone marrow transplant and not covered them. Ms. Ford subsequently received her chemotherapy, but she was still forced to forego the surgery, as she could not afford to pay for it. The hospital had since decided that they could not treat her on a self-paying basis.

Ms. Ford's pay from the IRS, where she faithfully worked for seventeen years, had run out; the donated sick-leave from her co-workers had also expired. With her chances of survival growing slimmer as each day passed, Ms. Ford began looking for other ways to finance her treatment. She enlisted the aid of an attorney—obviously a costly undertaking—to appeal the insurance company's decision. She applied for Medicaid, but the time involved in processing her application would make it too late for her scheduled transplant.

As Ms. Ford desperately pursued the possibility of obtaining treatment from other cancer centers, she received word that a public hospital had agreed to cover the cost of the bone marrow transplant—to be performed at Tulane Medical Center. After being repeatedly assured that the cost of the transplant would be covered, Ms. Ford dropped the appeal process with the insurance company, as well as all other efforts at trying to obtain treatment elsewhere. Tulane Medical Center then informed her that in order for the public hospital to cover the transplant, she would have to receive her mastectomy at the public hospital. The mastectomy and all other procedures were again canceled, further throwing off her treatment plan.

After rescheduling these procedures, Ms. Ford was then told that the public hospital had refused to cover the bone marrow transplant and that, furthermore, her insurance would not cover the mastectomy unless it was performed at Tulane Medical Center. With time running out, Ms. Ford had no choice but to reschedule again—and hope that somehow she could finance a bone marrow transplant. To be effective, the transplant would have to be undertaken within approximately three weeks of the mastectomy; an appeal of the insurance company's decision would take up to two months.

Just after Ms. Ford underwent her mastectomy, I became aware of her unbelievable plight. Literally shocked by the endeavor she had experienced, I contacted the Office of Personnel Management (OPM) in the hope of expediting the appeal process. Much to my dismay, I learned that Ms. Ford had once again been totally misled. Community Health Network, her insurance company, gave her the false hope that she could appeal their decision to OPM. In fact, OPM has no power to force a plan to finance a procedure which is excluded from coverage in the plan's contract—as bone marrow transplants plainly are. Ms. Ford was once again back where she started, and she had again wasted scarce time and energy which should have been spent fighting her cancer.

I was overjoyed to learn that last week, Ms. Ford's oncologist successfully persuaded the hospital to permit her treatment to continue. Apparently, Medicaid had agreed to cover the cost of the transplant. Although they have subsequently revoked this commitment, Ms. Ford's oncologist was still able to proceed with her treatment; the financial situation remains in flux.

I am here today on behalf of Ms. Ford . . . and countless women like her. The Federal Employees Health Benefits Program is failing miserably to address the needs of women with breast cancer. This disease, especially in an advanced diagnosis, is itself a horrendous proposition, but for women like Ms. Ford, everything boils down to money. In dealing with hospitals, the fatal illness becomes secondary, as a patient's focus must be on negotiating a good price to obtain parts of a treatment plan. It is truly abhorrent that our health care system, especially FEHBP, leaves women to bargain for life-saving treatment. Ms. Ford exemplifies the problem with our current health care system—a diligent, middle-class woman is forced into poverty in order to receive Medicaid coverage for her health care.

Many FEHBP policies, including Ms. Ford's, cover bone marrow transplants for testicular cancer and other diseases. OPM and the insurance companies claim that for breast cancer, this procedure is not covered because it is experimental—although many noted oncologists have maintained that the evidence supporting the use of bone marrow transplants as treatment for breast cancer is far superior to the evidence supporting the same treatment for testicular cancer.

The failure of insurance plans to cover bone marrow transplants for breast cancer patients is clearly discriminatory. Insurance plans reimburse for bone marrow transplants that are far more speculative in terms of their proven effectiveness—a practice which is inconsistent and blatantly unfair. It is unforgivable that women Federal employees with breast cancer are excluded from scientifically-advanced, effective treatment methods—a revamping of OPM's policy on this issue is long overdue.

Thank you for your consideration.

Ms. NORTON. You say that you hope we will move quickly to help remedy this situation. Congressman Lehman, I wonder if you and our other colleagues could indicate what you recommend, what action you recommend that the subcommittee take with respect to this issue?

Mrs. SCHROEDER. Basically, I think OPM should be told that I think this has come far enough along that it should be considered part of the treatment. I think you mentioned it even in your opening statement. And I particularly find it awful coming from a State where, if you are Blue Cross in the private sector, it is covered; if you are in the public sector, it is not. I think that is regressive and OPM should move on.

Mr. LEHMAN. I agree 100 percent. I think it is very clear that the current practice is discriminatory. There is ample scientific evidence on the other side not just to support the fact that this is effective, that it may be more effective than ones that they are already allowing.

And no one should be put in the position that the former constituent of mine was, literally going from handout to handout trying to find a way to finance this, when supposedly public employees are supposed to have a Cadillac insurance plan, the finest thing out there. To find out they'd be better off somewhere else is just terrible.

Mrs. VUCANOVICH. I think it is disappointing that the Federal employees are being treated this way. And I think when private insurers are taking care of them, it is just inexcusable. We have a lot of our constituents who say they want the same kind of plans we have. But when they get some of the details, they might say, no, thank you.

Mrs. SCHROEDER. Exactly.

Ms. NORTON. Each of you sits on committees and subcommittees where you have to gauge whether or not what the witness, particularly the Federal agency, for example, is telling you is the reason is, in fact, the reason. I am puzzled by the fact that there are insurance carriers that approve this treatment.

When you consider that insurance carriers, especially these days, may be the tightest-fisted folks around, the notion that there are carriers, apparently in significant numbers, that approve this treatment, at least in NCI treatment programs, raises the question for me, "why do you think OPM is holding back so long?"

Mrs. SCHROEDER. Madam Chair, I wish I knew. Obviously, you are going to have some experts here that know a whole lot more about what the medical community knows about the different treatments. But what's even more shocking to me is that OPM is demanding a higher standard for breast cancer treatment than they are for the other treatments that they already pay for.

You know what you are going to hear in the testimony. You are going to hear, well, we will pay for this as soon as NCI has come through with the whole study, and that the study shows that, indeed, this really works, except they never required that kind of standard for testicular cancer or for other cancers where they do allow this procedure.

So why do we have to have a higher standard than anybody else? It goes back to that old story we used to tell that men and women were treated the same in heaven. They all had to spell a word to get in. Men spelled "cat" and women had to spell "Czechoslovakia." It looks like OPM is using that on the issue.

Mrs. VUCANOVICH. I can't top that.

Ms. NORTON. There has been some suggestion, of course, that we could speculate that there is straight-out sex discrimination here. You would wonder if OPM would be foolish enough to engage in that—although there can be sex discrimination that is not entirely intentional but that is effectively sex discrimination.

There has been a suggestion that cost may be a factor here. I wonder if any of you have any comments on that?

Mrs. SCHROEDER. I think all of us have been round and round about that on mammograms. And the gentleman from Indiana pointed that out, our frustration with how they keep changing the guidelines on mammograms and so forth. And a lot of us suspect that everybody is looking at how do you make something fit into a certain cost standard. But I certainly hope that that is not the driving wedge, because I don't know how you put a cost on someone's life.

And I keep going back to the fact that I can't imagine anything worse than being in the position where you feel you or someone in your family's life is really in jeopardy and then to also think the entire financial security of the family is also in jeopardy and you have to determine whether to treat them or not on that basis. I can't believe it.

Mr. LEHMAN. Let me just say with respect to this case, which is what I am familiar with—and I got involved at the request of the family and called Mr. King at OPM. He returned all my phone calls and was very direct, had no problems with the personal relationship there at all, but made it very, very clear that there was no way.

In fact, one of the things Congresswoman Schroeder alluded to was brought up to me. It seemed to be the only way to get treatment here would be to get into an experimental situation. Imagine being in the position with life and death breast cancer. Your only hope, because you don't have the money to pay for it, is to get into an experimental situation where half get the treatment, half get a placebo, and you don't know which you are. I just can't imagine facing that kind of circumstance and putting somebody in that position borders on being inhuman.

Ms. NORTON. Congresswoman Vucanovich?

Mrs. VUCANOVICH. I just have to concur with both of my colleagues that, yes, a lot of these treatments are expensive. But, again, how important is your life? And why should our Federal employees be treated differently? I think that is my concern.

Ms. NORTON. If the expense here was for a treatment that had not shown such extraordinary promise and you could get an expensive treatment and still there was no significant statistical evidence that you would be aided, one could understand——

Mrs. SCHROEDER. Absolutely.

Ms. NORTON [continuing]. That you are not supposed to authorize large amounts where the information, the data simply don't confirm.

What is very troubling here is that this is a disease where we have not been able to find a fair number of treatments, very restrictive treatments. And here, for the first time, we have ample, more and more promising evidence coming from more and more studies, and yet for this disease, in the largest program in the country, we cannot get reimbursement. We need to get to the bottom of that today.

And your testimony leading off this hearing has been very important for setting the stage, and I very much appreciate your taking time out of the end-of-the-session busy schedules to come forward this morning.

May I ask Congresswoman Morella if she has any questions for you?

Mrs. MORELLA. Thank you.

I want to thank you for being here to testify to lead off this subcommittee.

Barbara, I particularly want to thank you because you have always been there any time something has come up with regard to women's health and breast cancer particularly, citing your own instance.

Mrs. VUCANOVICH. Thank you.

Mrs. MORELLA. Mr. Lehman, you are great to comment thoroughly about your constituent, and Pat has always been there with regard to women's health and women's issues.

I just find this a kind of a schizophrenic paranoia that is in the air. And I say that because not all insurance companies are paying in different regions for this in the private sector is what baffles me. The Federal government, of course, should be setting the tone.

You mentioned that there are certain areas where it is paid in the private sector; other areas where it is not. So I think this says something about not only OPM—and I look forward to questioning them on their testimony since they called this investigation—but also the fact that we should reign in these insurance companies, too, and make sure that consistently, throughout the country, that people do not have to resort to law cases if they, in fact, engage in this particular treatment or else go without the treatment.

So I find it arbitrary, capricious and all of those kind of points that come out in this. And I do believe that it will be very encouraging to hear from the experts and that we should be covering it in the Federal Employees Health Benefits Plan.

Mr. Myers has advised me that he can spell "Czechoslovakia." But I also want to compliment—I also want to compliment now that they have split—I want to compliment him on coming because he also has always been there when it comes to breast cancer.

My sister died of lymphoma, but she started off with breast cancer and there were no treatments available, so it spread. Thank you.

Thank you, Madam Chair.

Ms. NORTON. Thank you very much, Congresswoman Morella.

Congresswoman Byrne?

Ms. BYRNE. No, thank you.

Ms. NORTON. Congressman Myers. I am sorry.

Mr. MYERS. Not too many people on your left, but here I am. Thank you very much for your testimony.

I might add just one thing. Several have offered the excuse why it is not offered or considered by OPM is because it is still experimental. The fact is, all breast or all cancer treatment is experimental today. Different cancers, I have observed, respond differently to different treatment. Different chemos are used on different cancers. So we are still experimenting.

Some cancers respond to treatment rather simply, rather successfully. Others, the same treatment, look like the same stage, same location of the cancer of the body, but do not respond.

So there are so many questions. And the bottom line is about all the treatment is still experimental. Some are successful. Fortunately, more and more are becoming successful. But it still is experimental. So I don't think that is a very valid argument for why we don't provide it. There may be other reasons. I am anxious to find out.

Thank you for your testimony.

Mrs. SCHROEDER. Thank you.

Ms. NORTON. Thank you Congresswoman Vucanovich, Congressman Lehman and Congresswoman Schroeder.

May I ask panel two to come forward? These are survivors of breast cancer: Ms. Bonnie Reger, Ms. Renay McCarty, Mr. and Mrs. Ed McKulsky, and Miss Donna Rogers.

STATEMENTS OF BONNIE REGER; RENAY FRANCE McCARTY; MR. AND MRS. ED McKULSKY; AND DONNA K. ROGERS

Ms. NORTON. We will begin with Ms. Reger.

Ms. REGER. Pardon me?

Ms. NORTON. Actually, you can begin in any order you like.

Ms. REGER. I will go first, if that is all right.

Ms. NORTON. Thank you.

Ms. REGER. Thank you, Madam Chair, for the opportunity to express my concern over the lack of coverage of high-dose chemotherapy with autologous bone marrow transplant as a treatment for breast cancer under the Federal Employees Benefits Program. Having had the treatment last November, I can sit before you and honestly say that I have no reservation with regard to that treatment, and I strongly recommend coverage of the treatment in the Federal Employees Health Benefits Program.

I have had high option Blue Cross/Blue Shield under the Federal Employees Health Benefits Program for 23 years, my entire Federal career. I have had breast cancer for 14 years. In 1980, I had a mastectomy with no further treatment. In 1983—and I—that has to be corrected on my handout. I accidentally said 1980. In 1983, there was evidence of metastasis to bone. I was told by two oncologists to wrap things up, that at most I would have two and a half years on a hormone treatment of the breast cancer.

The hormone treatment was initiated with the drug Tamoxifan, and the reason I mention this is that in 1983, Tamoxifan was considered an experimental drug. That drug kept me disease-free for six years. It took nine years for the hormone treatment to run its course and, finally, just fail in 1992.

In 1992, I knew that I either wanted to die or I wanted a bone marrow transplant. It took until 1993 to finally become an acceptable candidate for a bone marrow transplant at Emory University Hospital. That is in 1993, I became a candidate at Emory, and that is when I discovered that the entire Federal system and Blue Cross/Blue Shield failed me. I was denied coverage for the bone marrow transplant.

The transplant was obtained with no thanks to OPM or Blue Cross/Blue Shield. Blue Cross/Blue Shield, in 1993, specifically excluded bone marrow transplant procedures for breast cancer, and the U.S. Office of Personnel Management did not have and still does not have a policy that will cover the procedure for breast cancer.

I had fallen through the cracks of this system, and I was faced with having to come up with $150,000 myself for treatment. Others need it and are sitting on a time bomb. And that is why I am here today. Coverage is overdue. With your help, we should be able to get it into the Federal Employees Benefits Program.

I would like to make one comment before I close. Everybody is talking about NCI trials. Very few people qualify for NCI trials. They can run on from now until eternity before the trials ever end. I was never eligible for that treatment, and today I feel perfectly normal and test results prove that I am perfectly normal as a result of the bone marrow transplant.

Thank you.

Ms. NORTON. Thank you very much.

[The prepared statement of Ms. Reger follows:]

PREPARED STATEMENT OF BONNIE REGER

Thank you for the opportunity to express my concern over the lack of coverage for high-dose chemotherapy with autologous bone marrow transplant (HDC/ABMT) as a treatment for breast cancer under the Federal Employees Health Benefits Program (FEHBP). Having had the treatment in late November of 1993 at Emory University Hospital, I can honestly say that I would not hesitate to go through the procedure to feel as well as I do now. I feel like a new person as a result of the treatment. Based on my good experience I highly recommend coverage of HDC/ABMT for breast cancer in the FEHBP.

Personal history: joined USDA, ARS in 1971; enrolled in the FEHBP high option Blue Cross/Blue Shield (BC/BS) since 1971; diagnosed with breast cancer in 1980; evidence of metastasis to bone in 1980, hormone treatment from 1983 to 1992 [Tamoxifen, then experiental, kept me disease free for six years]; 1992 hormone treatment no longer effective, left with chemotherapy and potentially HDC/ABMT; and July 1993 taxol had dramatically improved my situation, became a candidate for HDC/ABMT and was scheduled for early September. Treatment was delayed until late November of 1993 because of BC/BS's preadmission denial of treatment and loss of my appeals to BC/BS and FEHBP. Knowing first hand the feeling of having a short window of opportunity for benefit from HDC/ABMT, not being eligible for one of the BC/BS trial studies (where you have 50/50 chance of obtaining HDC/ABMT), the uncertainty of BC/BS continued coverage for taxol treatments (each admission was preceded with advice from BC/BS that preadmission did not automatically mean payment), and facing the impossibility of personally paying for the procedure I am here to say on behalf of others in that dilemma that it was unconscionable of FEHBP to have negotiated policies in 1993 excluding this treatment (continues to date), leaving federal employees with preexisting or newly diagnosed breat cancer out on a limb. In addition, inclusion of BMT for testicular cancer when trial studies seem to indicate lack of benefit and the specific exclusion of HDC/ABMT for breast cancer appears to be discriminatory.

The issue of sex discrimination will be decided in Federal Court; I am suing BC/BS, U.S. OPM, and USDA. I am after a change in policy and legal fees (no personal financial gain). My obligation is twofold: (1) To Emory; agreed to continue the court case at my expense in exchange for the treatment; and (2) To others who are either in or may eventually be in the dilemma in which I found myself in August of 1993.

It is worth pointing out that insurance policies covering HDC/ABMT for breast cancer can be obtained in Colorado and Virginia unless of course you are federally employed and are under the FEHBP. Also, is there a better way of doing business? In 1993 the University of Georgia (UGA) being self-insured ordered BC/BS to pay for an employee's HDC/ABMT for breast cancer "out of contract." Apparently UGA's financial pool is large enough to pay for uncovered procedures even though UGA employees pay less than federal employees for healthcare. Wouldn't the federal government have considerably more money to operate similarly?

Ms. NORTON. Yes. Who wants to speak next?

Ms. MCCARTY. Thank you.

My name is Renay France McCarty, and I have been covered by the Federal employees health plan program since mid–1980, and today, Madam Chairman, I would like to request the committee require all Federal plans cover autologous bone marrow bone for breast cancer. This could be accomplished by making the treatment reasonable and a necessary medical expense under each plan or making it available as a supplemental benefit which an employee can elect and pay for at an additional cost.

However, should this committee decide otherwise, then I have two suggestions. The first is that all plans covering the treatment provide—not covering the treatment provide in bold and conspicuous manner on the front of its brochures the following statement: Breast cancer affects nearly one of nine women in the United States. For some persons, a bone marrow transplant has been shown to be effective treatment for breast cancer. Note, however, this plan does not cover bone marrow transplants for breast cancer.

The second suggestion, in the alternative, is that the committee request the appropriate Federal agency to undertake an epidemiological study to compare the ratio of the number of Federal employees requesting and receiving coverage of this treatment under Federal plans to the number requesting and receiving coverage of this treatment under comparable private plans. In my view, this data will demonstrate that disparate treatment now exists between Federal employees and private-sector employees under comparable health plans. This has been my experience.

In the early 1980's, physicians began treating advanced cancer—advanced breast cancer with bone marrow transplants. As you know, most issuers refused to pay for this procedure, calling it experimental. Hospitals would only admit you if you agreed—if the insurer agreed to pay. As a result, most of these patients, while combatting cancer and facing their mortality in a forceful way and at a very intimate moment, also contended with financing the treatment themselves, usually at a cost ranging between 150 to $200,000.

Some financed the treatment from personal resources, if wealthy. Some financed this treatment through community fund-raisers. Some, with the assistance of hospitals, obtained an injunction under which the insurer paid the hospital up front with the issue of coverage being decided after treatment had been provided. And some, those not so strong in their constitution, gave up this onerous and strenuous battle for this treatment and, with that, often their lives.

In 1989, while yet in my 30s, I developed breast cancer. I had a recurrence in 1989 and a second recurrence in 1990. In April of 1991, my physicians advised me to obtain a bone marrow transplant within two months.

I went to the University of Chicago, Illinois Hospital Center, trying to obtain this treatment through my carrier at that time, Blue Cross/Blue Shield. I received no word about coverage of this treatment for nearly three weeks. My option at that time was to either have my insurer agree to pay or I would have to pay $200,000 up front. I contacted John Hopkins University, also Georgetown University with the same result.

Fortunately, it was just by stroke of luck that I went to Sloan–Kettering Hospital in New York where they agreed to admit me without having the precertification from the insurer or the up-front payment of $200,000.

Before being admitted into Sloan, I notified Blue Cross by phone of the impending treatment and obtained oral certification. Subsequently, Blue Cross sent me a letter informing me that it needed more information before it could certify that coverage. Letters went back and forth between Sloan and Blue Cross without Blue Cross giving an answer to the certification.

Because I needed treatment quickly, I proceeded on. I received high-dose chemotherapy with stem cell infusion, technically not a bone marrow transplant, without the certification or the repayment. I agreed with Sloan, however, that I would bring suit to recover any payments should Blue Cross not provide it. I remained hospitalized at Sloan for 42 days, from August 5 to September 13, 1991.

Finally, in 1992, Blue Cross informed me that the procedure could have been performed on an outpatient basis and denied approximately $80,000 of medical cost. It did pay for the procedures that could have been performed on an outpatient basis. At that time, no reputable medical institution in the United States provided bone marrow transplants on an outpatient basis. It was an incredible explanation for the denial of benefits.

Under my agreement with Sloan, I had to bring action against Blue Cross to pay for that remaining $80,000. Federal employees can only sue after appealing with the Office of Personnel Management. I did so. OPM denied my appeal in favor of Blue Cross. This action effectively stripped me of any legal redress because no court has ever reversed OPM on a question of fact in the absence of abuse.

With respect to private-sector plans, however, every court case involving this issue has decided in favor of the patient-plaintiff.

The above facts clearly demonstrate that my status as a Federal employee and OPM's actions precluded my obtaining full coverage of my medical and legal costs in a fashion similar to private-sector employees with comparable coverage.

From August 5 to September 13, 1991, three women received high-dose chemotherapy with stem cell infusion at Sloan. The first, a homemaker, had her treatment fully paid by Blue Cross under her husband's private-sector plan. The second, who was unemployed and originally from Norway, had her treatment fully paid by Medicare. I was the third, gainfully employed with the Federal government and with health insurance. I still owe nearly $80,000 in medical costs to Sloan-Kettering on August 11, 1994. I believe that something is wrong with this picture.

Thank you.

Ms. NORTON. Thank you very much.

[The prepared statement of Ms. McCarty follows:]

PREPARED STATEMENT OF RENAY FRANCE MCCARTY

My name is Renay France McCarty, and since mid-1980 to the present, I have been a Federal employee, covered by a Federal Employees Health Benefit Plan.

My testimony today requests that the Committee require all Federal Employees Health Benefit Plans to cover autologous bone marrow transplants for breast cancer. This could be accomplished by making the treatment a reasonable and necessary medical expense under each plan or by making it available as a supplemental benefit which an employee could elect at an additional cost, borne in full or in part by the electing employee.

Should this Committee decide otherwise, then I have two suggestions. The first is that all plans not covering the treatment provide in a bold and conspicuous manner on the front of its brochures the following statement—breast cancer affects nearly one of nine women in the United States. For some persons, a bone marrow transplant has been shown to be effective treatment for breast cancer. Note, however, this plan does not cover bone marrow transplants for breast cancer.

The second suggestion is that the Committee request the appropriate Federal agency to undertake an epidemiological study to compare the ratio of the number of Federal employees requesting and receiving coverage of this treatment under Federal plans to the number requesting and receiving coverage of this treatment under comparable private plans. In my view this data will demonstrate that disparate treatment now exists between Federal employees and private-sector employees under comparable health plans. This has been my experience.

In the early 80's physicians began treating advanced breast cancer patients with bone marrow transplants. Most insurers denied coverage of the procedure, calling it "experimental." Hospitals would not admit you unless the insurer agreed to pay. As a result, these patients, while combatting cancer and facing their mortality in a very intimate way, also contended with financing the treatment themselves, usually at a cost ranging between $150,000 to $200,000.

Some financed the treatment from personal resources, if lucky and wealthy; some financed the treatment through community fund raisers; some, with the assistance of the hospital, obtained an injunction under which the insurer paid the hospital up-front with the issue of coverage being decided after treatment had been provided; and some, those not so strong in constitution, gave up the battle for this treatment and with that, often their lives.

In 1988, while yet in my 30's, I developed breast cancer. I had a recurrence in 1989, and a second recurrence in 1990. In April of 1991, my physicians advised me to obtain a bone marrow transplant by July of that year.

I went to the University of Chicago seeking treatment, which required a certification of payment by my insurer or $200,000 up-front. The hospital contacted the Chicago area Federal Employees Program for Blue Cross/Blue Shield (BC/BS), my insurer, at the time. For nearly three weeks, we received no definitive answer from BC/BS. Then I went to Johns Hopkins and Georgetown University Hospitals; both required the same certification or up-front payment. Fortunately, Sloan Kettering Hospital admitted me without requiring either, provided that I file suit against BC/BS in the event of its nonpayment.

Before being admitted into Sloan, I notified BC/BS by phone of the impending treatment and obtained oral certification. Subsequently, BC/BS sent me a letter informing me that it needed more information before it could certify the coverage. Letters went back and forth between Sloan and BC/BS without BC/BS giving an answer as to certification. Because I needed treatment quickly, I proceeded with treatment at Sloan, high dose chemotherapy with stem cell infusion—technically not a bone marrow transplant—without the certication or prepayment. I remained hospitalized at Sloan for 42 days, from August 5 to September 13, 1991.

Finally, in 1992, BC/BC informed me that the procedure could have been performed on an out-patient basis and denied approximately $80,000 of medical costs. (It did pay for the procedures that could have been performed on an out-patient basis). At that time, no reputable medical institution in the United States provided bone morrow transplants on an out-patient basis. It was an incredible explanation for the denial of benefits.

Meanwhile, during my hospitalization, a woman in an adjacent room at Sloan, with identical recurrent breast cancer, receiving identical treatment, and covered by BS/BS under comparable contract provisions with a private employer, received nearly $350,000 of covered treatment.

Under my agreement with Slaon, I had to bring action against BC/BS to pay the remaining $80,000. Federal employees can only sue after filing an appeal with the Office of Personnel Management (OPM). I appealed to OPM, which decided in favor of BC/BS. This action effectively stripped me of any legal redress because no Court had reversed OPM on a question of fact, in the absence of abuse.

With respect to private-sector plans, however, every court case involving this issue has been decided in favor of the patient-plaintiff. Furthermore, in many of these cases, the plaintiff recovered attorneys' fees as well. Being precluded from bringing action, I do not know whether I could have recovered any legal costs. One attorney, assisting me in appealing with OPM, requested a $5,000 retainer.

The above facts clearly demonstrate that my status as a Federal employee and OPM's actions precluded my obtaining full coverage of medical and legal costs in a fashion similar to private-sector employees with comparable coverage.

From August 5 to September 13, 1991, three women received high dose chemotherapy with stem cell infusion at Sloan. The first, a homemaker, had her treatment fully paid by BC/BS under her husband's private-sector plan. The second, who was unemployed and originally from Norway, had her treatment fully paid by Medicaid. I was the third, gainfully employed with the Federal Government and with health insurance. I still owe nearly $80,000 in medical costs to Sloan Kettering on August 11, 1994. I believe that something is wrong with this picture.

Thank you for allowing me to testify on this very important health issue. I will be happy to answer your questions and to provide you with any additional documentation concerning this testimony.

Ms. NORTON. Yes.

Mrs. CATHARINE MCKULSKY. Madam Chair and other Members, I am Catharine McKulsky. I am a bone marrow transplant survivor.

Ms. NORTON. Can you move the microphone?

Mrs. CATHARINE McKULSKY. Three and a half years ago, I was diagnosed with breast cancer. At that time, my two boys, Edward and Matthew, were five and six years old. Because I was able to have a bone marrow transplant, I am alive and cancer free today. If I had not been able to have the transplant, I probably would not have seen my 40th birthday, and my children, Edward and Matthew, would have had to grow up without a mother.

The decision to have a bone marrow transplant was a difficult decision, but once I decided to do it, and realized that it was really my only option, I was fully committed. However, both my insurance company and the Office of Personnel Management (OPM), were not committed.

When I began my protocol with Duke University, I knew that in order to have my bone marrow harvested, I had to have either my insurance company approval or else $90,000 in cash. One week prior to my bone marrow harvesting, I received a phone call at 3:00 in the afternoon. It was my husband, and he told me that the insurance company denied me. I was devastated. I fell to the floor. I literally felt like someone had kicked me in the stomach.

Tears were streaming down my face, and my children ran over to me and asked me, mommy, what's wrong? What happened? How do you tell a five and a six-year-old child that their mother is not worth $90,000? How do you tell a five and six-year-old child that a group of people, people that don't even know their mother, met in a boardroom and decided that their mother doesn't deserve to have the chance to live?

It was only after my husband and I initiated litigation that our insurance company decided to pay the majority of the cost for the transplant. But many women are not as fortunate as I was. And a woman this past year, I think, exemplifies this, Ms. Marlene Fox, in California.

She exemplifies how the denial and the delay can be deadly. Her insurance company denied her, and because she and her family had to go out and raise funds—women often do this through contributions, mortgaging their homes and or liquidating their whole life's savings. And because of the delay, she was not able to get the bone marrow transplant in a timely fashion and she died.

I pray that more women don't have to die before insurance companies and before OPM are held accountable. I pray that women in the future don't have to turn to their children and say, yes, in the United States of America, there is a treatment that could possibly cure your mother, but because of an insurance company policy or because of OPM policy, your mother has been denied treatment and your mother doesn't get the chance to live.

Thank you.

Ms. NORTON. Thank you.

[The prepared statement of Mrs. McKulsky follows:]

PREPARED STATEMENT OF CATHARINE McKULSKY

I am a bone marrow transplant survivor. Three and a half years ago, when I was thirty-eight years old, I was diagnosed with breast cancer. My two boys Eddie and Matthew were five and six years old. Because I was able to have an analogous bone marrow transplant, I am alive and cancer free today. Had it not been for the transplant, I probably would not have lived to see my fortieth birthday and my young children would have had to grow up without a mother.

Three and a half years ago, I had to not only cope with the devastation of being diagnosed with breast cancer, but I had to overcome difficulties within the medical field, and with my health insurance company and the Office of Personnel Management (OPM). The day before my appointment with an oncologist a woman called me who had the same oncologist. She had been diagnosed with ten positive lymph nodes. I was diagnosed with eighteen. She told me that on her first visit to the oncologist, he immediately told her that he would give her standard chemotherapy but that in six months after the chemo she would have a recurrence. Needless to say, six months after her chemotherapy she had a recurrence.

Neither at the time of her recurrence, nor during her first visit with the oncologist did he offer her the option of a bone marrow transplant. Unfortunately, within a year she died. I am thankful to her for the phone call because after talking to her, I canceled my appointment with that oncologist and found an oncologist who believed in treating breast cancer aggressively.

I have since come to realize that too many oncologists believe that advanced breast cancer is not curable and therefore only give minimal treatment. It concerns me that there are physicians out there that either through ignorance or through misinformation do not offer women, who need aggressive treatment, the option of a bone marrow transplant.

Besides uninformed oncologists, women who need bone marrow transplants have an additional obstacle—insurance coverage, and in my case, OPM. Though the decision to have a bone marrow transplant was difficult, once I decided it was my best option, I was fully committed. However my insurance company and OPM were not committed.

I knew that prior to having my bone marrow harvested I needed either my insurance company's approval or ninety-thousand dollars in cash. One week prior to my bone marrow harvesting, I received a phone call at three o'clock on a Friday afternoon. My husband told me the insurance company had denied me. I fell to the floor. I literally felt like someone had kicked me in the stomach. Tears were streaming down my face. Eddie and Matt came running over to me and asked "Mommy what's wrong?"

How do you tell a five and six year old child that their mommy isn't worth ninety-thousand dollars?

How do you tell a five and six year old child that a group of people, who do not even know their mommy, met in a board room and decided that their mommy does not get a chance to live.

After I and my husband initiated litigation, I was fortunate that my insurance company covered most of the costs for this successful treatment. However many women are not as fortunate as I was. For these women, this means that they and their families have to raise the funds through contributions, mortgaging homes, and/or liquidating all their life savings before the women are able to receive care.

As exemplified by Nelene Fox in California, too frequently this delay is deadly. Her insurance company denied her coverage, and because of the delay caused by having to raise money, she was unable to receive a bone marrow transplant in a timely manner and died. The California court held the insurance company negligent and awarded the family a considerable amount of money.

I pray more women do not have to die before the insurance companies and OPM are held accountable. I pray that women in the future do not have to explain to their children that yes in the United States of America there is treatment available that could cure your mother but because of an insurance company and OPM's policy your mommy was denied treatment and does not get a chance to live.

Mr. EDWARD MCKULSKY. Madam Chair, committee members, ladies and gentlemen, you have a copy of my statement. I would just like to make a few more comments.

The one thing that is most important is our oncologist, our plan doctor, recommended this form of treatment. He worked for the insurance company, basically. And when he made the recommendation to us, we accepted it, of course, because it was about an 80 percent better chance that my wife was going to live through this life-threatening illness.

The plan turned against us, as my wife mentioned. We have appealed to the insurance company, to OPM and even to the First Lady to try to get them to address this problem.

Last September, my wife and I attended a function at the White House in the Rose Garden. We represented 700,000 letters that were sent there. And it was a very good experience for us.

The thing that I noticed most is that the President, when he had an opportunity to speak, was saying that he wanted a more comprehensive and equitable health system for everyone, but he also said that it would be more costly for less coverage. And I became mesmerized by that statement. It was like being on a roller coaster, listening to some of the comments that were made by everyone.

As an example, what was just said here today is that they are trying to raise the age of mammograms to women over 50 years old and require one every two years. That is a good example of what I am trying to say. In Virginia, we finally got a law passed where we are going to have bone marrow transplants for breast cancer, but the Federal employees apparently are going to be excluded.

What I am trying to do now is to get people to realize that in the Federal government we have had a kind of contradictory policy for some time. That is, the Department of Health and Human Services will give a bone marrow transplant to anyone that is entitled to veterans benefits or to Medicaid, and they have been doing that for some time.

And I just find it really ironic and unique that in the Federal government we can have one department that is against it and another department that supports it. We should be able to get together on this idea.

Another thing is, that they keep trying to say that this is investigational and experimental. How can it be investigational and experimental when at Duke University, over the last 10 years or more, they treated over 800 women and more than 72 percent are alive and some of them past 10 years? The median of this group is six years.

I just do not agree with all the experts that want to keep categorizing this as experimental and investigational when you have those kinds of results. You will see in a lot of the statements that are against bone marrow transplant, that they say that there is no consensus. But I think if anyone ever contacted the oncologists and asked them the majority, 51 percent, what they would be for, I think you would find that they would recommend a bone marrow transplant for breast cancer.

I have no further comment.

Ms. NORTON. Thank you.

[The prepared statement of Mr. McKulsky follows:]

PREPARED STATEMENT OF EDWARD MCKULSKY

In September 1993, my wife and I, and about 100 other citizens, were invited to the White House Rose Garden to meet with the President, and Mrs. Clinton, Vice-President, and Mrs. Gore. We were representing the 700,000 that had written to Mrs. Clinton's task force. The President presented the health problems that we had experienced, as examples, of the 700,000 letters sent in. Everyone in attendance appreciated his effort.

During the President's presentation, he said he wanted a more comprehensive and equitable health system. He also said it would be more costly, for less coverage. While feeling mesmerized, I began to worry about all those who failed to obtain catastrophic coverage from insurance companies and the Office of Personnel Management (OPM) for breast cancer treatment, and now the President just said, we are going to have less coverage (to cover more people). Many have needlessly died of breast cancer, and it appears, will continue under the President's new program.

When I wrote to Mrs. Clinton, I told her that I had written to the Office of Personnel Management, and asked them to fix a disparate and contradictory health policy, affecting everyone covered under the Federal Employees Health Benefits Plans (FEHBP), without success.

Presently, nearly 100 percent of the health plans available to federal employees will not pay for a bone marrow transplant for breast cancer, and for many other forms of cancer, as well. OPM, who manages the federal system, allows most insurance companies including the largest, Blue Cross-Blue Shield, to deny this coverage, based on that it is experimental and investigational, or that it is not covered under the FEHBP.

However, if you qualify for Medicaid or Veterans Benefits, the Department of Health and Human Services, will pay with taxpayers money for this treatment.

How can one department of government (OPM) allow insurance companies to consider it as experimental and investigational treatment, when the Department of Health and Human Services, will pay for it. This is contradictory. It would be better for the government to fix this problem first, as an example of an equitable and comprehensive plan, before trying to fix the country's health system.

This current policy is ridiculous. Over 70 percent of the patients (over 800) that have had this treatment at Duke University Medical Center during the past 10 years, are still alive. These survivors had a three day reunion in Washington, DC, in October 1993, and met with many members of Congress.

Ms. NORTON. Yes.

Ms. ROGERS. Madam Chairman, I am Donna Rogers. I am from Denver, Colorado.

I am also a breast cancer survivor, but I have had to fight more than just my disease. I have had to battle the Office of Personnel Management and my insurance company in order to receive this lifesaving procedure.

In April 1990, I found a lump in my right breast. It was malignant. I had a lumpectomy and an axilliary node dissection and found that the cancer had spread beyond the lymph nodes, so I was treated with the standard protocol of three chemotherapies, 35 radiation treatments and then three more chemotherapies. This was all done under the Kaiser Health Care system. I was with a different employer at that time.

In June 1991, I took a position with the Resolution Trust Corporation in Denver in their Legal Division. And because I was on an annual, renewable contract, I had immediate coverage under the FDIC/RTC health care program, and in filling out my health forms, I fully disclosed that I had been previously treated for breast cancer and that I was, in fact, still receiving periodic checkups but otherwise in good health.

A persistent pain in my left hip sent me to the doctor in June of 1992, and, after several tests, it was determined that my breast cancer had reoccurred in the bone. Hormone therapy was tried, but it did not retard the progression of the disease.

On October 2, 1992, I sat in my oncologist's office and was told the following words: I have a treatment—you have a treatment choice to make. You can either have chemotherapy until your death in approximately 24 months, or you can have a bone marrow transplant. Those words don't really register quite accurately when someone tells you that.

But sitting in a stunned state, I thought, well, two years, I am not really quite through with living. Maybe I will investigate the bone marrow, which I did, and felt very sure that this was the treatment I wanted.

I very carefully read my employee benefits booklet before proceeding with the transplant because I wanted to make sure that it was covered. And there is no language in my benefits booklet about any kind of transplant, whether or not it is covered, or what possible restrictions there might be. So I proceeded to take the tests necessary to qualify for a bone marrow transplant and was accepted as a candidate under the University of Colorado Hospital program.

I knew I would need preapproval for the hospitalization part of the transplant, but I didn't anticipate too much trouble because they had already covered all my other treatments and all my checkups. Any amount of chemotherapy or treatments seem like they would be covered.

I had already started my induction chemotherapy for the transplant in November of 1992 when I received my denial letter from Blue Cross. Naturally, I was very upset. I knew that this induction chemotherapy program was very strenuous and I probably wouldn't have the strength and energy necessary to raise the money myself. I decided that I would write a letter requesting reconsideration of my case.

Then the second denial letter came, and it mentioned an amendment to the contract between the FDIC/RTC and Blue Cross/Blue Shield which specifically said that bone marrow transplant was not covered for breast cancer.

I called my administration officer at the Denver office and requested a copy of the contract and this amendment and was told that they didn't have that contract or the amendment in Denver. I would have to call OPM in Washington.

I had difficulty reaching them. I called several times a day for a week and then sent many electronic mails before I received a response. The person at OPM said, well, the contract is too large. We can't send that to you. But I will fax you a copy of the amendment which denies your coverage.

Well, they faxed four out of the five pages, omitting to send a page that I very much needed. It took another dozen phone calls and electronic mails before the missing page was finally faxed to me.

I had a local attorney look over my benefits booklet and the amendment and he didn't feel that I had a case, so I said, well, I guess I will go ahead with the induction chemotherapy and see if that might do some good, because it is more intense than standard protocol.

But I felt that at this kind of point in one's life—it is difficult, at best, to face the fact that your cancer has reoccurred, that your life expectancy is shortened and death stares you squarely in the face. And then, at the same time, you have got to take on the job of fighting for your survival with doctors, hospitals, chemicals, not to mention insurance companies and attorneys while you are feeling very ill.

I could not continue work, so I took leave without pay. I just plain did not have the energy and resources to start a fund-raising project for myself in the time period allotted.

My chemo cycles continued from November of 1992 through February of 1993, and it was then that I learned that a New Jersey attorney, Arlene Groch, had successfully fought several Blue Cross cases for other Federal employees. And I contacted her, and she looked over my benefits booklet and denial letters and felt maybe we would have a chance.

So now I got to start—to search for funds for legal fees. I couldn't put a second mortgage on my home because I was only working part-time and would not qualify. Finally, I borrowed money from friends and relatives so we could proceed with the case, and we filed suit on March 29, 1993.

Then the waiting began. This was even more stressful than the treatment that I had been undergoing, because time was a critical factor. I needed to receive an answer by April 9, 1993 in order to avoid having another induction treatment.

Finally, Blue Cross/Blue Shield consented to pay for my transplant on the morning of April 9. I was overjoyed. At the same time, it was a bittersweet victory. I felt such frustration and anger for having to go through all the stress of filing a lawsuit and the humiliating task of borrowing monies that I did not know how I would pay back. I would probably have to sell my home in order to pay off these debts. I did not feel that I should have had to deal with this extra worry and anxiety. The cancer was enough.

Fortunately for me, I received the treatment, and today I am cancer free. It is been 16 months since my transplant, and I am again in good health and have returned to work.

It is my contention that the insurance company would have paid as much money for the standard protocol of doctors, chemotherapy, home health care and/or hospice for the 24 months of my predicted life expectancy as it paid for my bone marrow transplant.

It is my understanding that it costs about $60,000 a year for treatment of a cancer patient. When you consider that a transplant these days is about 120,000 to 130,000, it seems to me much more beneficial to have the insurance companies and OPM agree to provide that kind of service to Federal employees. And they just might come out like I did, alive and well, and they wouldn't become another death statistic.

Today, I am a very active member of the Colorado Breast Cancer Coalition. I talk to and assist other breast cancer patients in seeking support and information on breast cancer and bone marrow transplant. I hope that other women can profit from my experience and not have to go through the same ordeal I did in order to receive the necessary medical treatment.

Thank you.

[The prepared statement of Ms. Rogers follows:]

PREPARED STATEMENT OF DONNA K. ROGERS

I am a breast cancer survivor, but I have had to fight more than just my disease. I have had to battle with personnel management and my insurance company in order to receive a life saving procedure.

In April, 1990, I found a lump in my right breast. A biopsy showed breast cancer. I had a lumpectomy and axilliary node dissection. Six out of nineteen nodes were positive for breast cancer, so I had three chemotherapies of a standard protocol, 35 radiation treatments, and 3 more chemotherapies. As of October, 1990, I was disease free. All of this treatment was done under the Kaiser Permanente Health Care system provided by my employer, Centennial Engineering.

In June, 1991, I took a position with RTC in Denver in the Legal Division. Because I was on an annual, renewable contract, I received immediate benefits under the FDIC/RTC health care program. In filling out my health forms I fully disclosed my previous treatment for breast cancer and the fact that I was still receiving periodic checkups. Otherwise I was in good health.

A persistent pain in my left hip sent me to the doctor in June, 1992, and after several tests it was determined that my breast cancer had reoccurred in the bone. Hormone therapy was tried but it did not retard the progression of the cancer.

On October 2, 1992, my oncologist informed me that I had a treatment choice to make. I could take chemotherapy until my death in approximately 24 months or I could have a bone marrow transplant.

After doing some research about bone marrow transplant, I decided that this was the treatment I wanted. I then carefully read my employee health benefits booklet from Blue Cross/Blue Shield. I did not find any information about treatments or transplants not being covered. I proceeded to take all the tests necessary to qualify for being bone marrow transplant candidate and was accepted to the University of Colorado program.

I knew that I would need to have pre-approval from Blue Cross/Blue Shield for the hospitalization required for the transplant. Previous to this request, I had not had any problems with insurance covering my treatments and checkups. I had already started my induction chemotherapy in November, 1992, when I received a letter from Blue Cross denying coverage for my bone marrow transplant. Naturally I was very upset. I knew that I would not have the strength or the energy to raise the monies necessary to pay for the treatment myself so I wrote a letter to the Blue Cross requesting a reconsideration of my case.

I received a second denial from the insurance company and this second denial letter mentioned an amendment to the insurance contract which specifically said that bone marrow transplant was not covered for breast cancer. I called my administration officer at work and requested a copy of the Blue Cross contract and the amendment. I was told that there was no copy of this contract in the Denver office. I would have to request these items from Office of Personnel Management in Washington, D.C. I called several times a day for a week and sent three electronic mails before I received a response. The person at OPM said that the contact was too large to send to me, but I could get a copy of the amendment which denied coverage. I was faxed four out of five pages of the amendment, the page which was omitted was the one I needed. It took another dozen phone calls and electronic mails before the missing page was finally faxed.

I had a local attorney look over the benefits booklet and the amendment and he felt that I did not have a case, so I decided not to pursue the matter. I hoped that the induction chemotherapy would possibly put me into remission since the chances for a transplant did not look good. It is difficult at best to handle the fact that your cancer has reoccurred, your life expectancy is shortened and death stares you squarely in the face. Then at the same time you must take on the job of fighting for your survival with doctors, hospitals, chemicals, not to mention the insurance company and attorneys, while being very ill. Since I was feeling the side effects of the rigorous induction chemo, I took a leave without pay from work. I did not have the energy or resources to start a fund raising project for myself. Besides I felt that my insurance should cover this procedure. I was too tired, too ill and too depressed to continue this fight.

My chemo cycles continued from November, 1992, until February, 1993. I learned that a New Jersey attorney, Arlene Groch, had successfully fought Blue Cross for other federal employees, and I decided to contact her to see what she thought about my case. Ms. Groch reviewed the benefit booklet and denial letters I sent her and she felt we had a good chance of being able to sue for treatment.

I began to search for funds to pay for the legal fees. A second mortgage on my house was out of the question because I was only working parttime and could not qualify for any additional payments. I still was not strong enough to launch a fund raising campaign. Finally I borrowed money from friends and relatives so we could proceed with the case. The suit was filed on March 29, 1993, and then the waiting began. This was even more stressful. . .waiting to hear if I would be given a chance to live. Time was a crucial factor as I needed to receive the answer by April 9, 1993, in order to avoid having another induction chemo treatment.

Finally Blue Cross/Blue Shield consented to pay for my transplant on the morning of April 9, 1993. I was overjoyed! At the same time it was bittersweet victory. I had felt such frustration and anger for having to go through all the stress of filing the lawsuit and the humiliating task of borrowing monies that I did not know how I would pay back. I would possibly have to sell my home in order to pay off these debts. I did not feel that I should have had to deal with all of this extra worry and anxiety. . . .the cancer was enough to deal with.

Fortunately for me, I received my treatment and today I am cancer free. It has been 16 months since my transplant. I am again in good health and have returned to work.

It is my contention that the insurance company would have paid as much money for the standard protocol of doctors, chemotherapy, home health care and/or Hospice for the 24 months of life expectancy as it paid for my bone marrow transplant. When all other treatments have failed, a bone marrow transplant becomes the only possible life saving procedure for many breast cancer patients. I do not feel that patients should be systematically denied a treatment that could save their lives. I am living proof that without this treatment I would not be speaking to you today. I would be just another breast cancer death statistic.

My experience was certainly enlightening to my fellow employees in the Denver office. It is more than a little scary to think that at any time you may be denied coverage for a treatment that could save your life, and you as an employee might not ever be aware of changes or amendments to your health insurance coverage. Employers should let their employees know exactly what is and what is not coveraged in their health insurance packages. Changes in benefits, either additions or deletions, must be communicated to all employees in a timely manner.

Today I am a very active member of the Colorado Breast Cancer Coalition. I talk to and assist other breast cancer patients seeking support and information about breast cancer and bone marrow transplant. I hope that other women can profit from my experience and not have to go through the same ordeal I experienced in order to receive the necessary medical treatment.

Ms. NORTON. The Members have to go to adjourn to vote. If you want to say anything before you go, I hope you will come back when OPM and NCI are before us.

Mrs. MORELLA. I just want to thank the panel. Very, very moving testimony. Thank you for coming. You are very courageous.

Did I hear Medicaid covers this?

Mr. EDWARD McKULSKY. Yes.

Ms. McCARTY. Yes.

Mr. EDWARD McKULSKY. I know the Health and Human Services Department will pay for it with taxpayers' money. But if you have an insurance plan under the Federal employees benefit plan, you don't get it.

Ms. ROGERS. If you're rich enough, you can go out and pay cash. That is fine. If you are a middle-class American, a working person like myself—I wasn't poor enough to receive the treatment under Medicaid without divesting myself of my home and all of my possessions.

Ms. NORTON. Thank you very much. Because I am a Delegate, there are about ninety-five percent of matters to vote on. The one I am most pleased not to have to vote on is the journal.

Mr. MYERS. Will you continue then?

Ms. NORTON. Yes, I will continue and hope you will come back.

In order to have this treatment, does the oncologist have to recommend that the treatment be administered? I am sorry—in your cases, I should ask.

Mr. EDWARD McKULSKY. In my wife's situation, when we went to the oncologist, because she had 18 of 22 lymph nodes involved, he said anything over 10 is a high risk for reoccurrence. And there was only one form of treatment that he recommended, and that was the ABMT. And it took us about 30 minutes to agree with his recommendation. And then we had to submit it and go down to Duke and be evaluated.

And my wife passed the pretest, so to speak, but the insurance company denied us. And then we went through the appeal process and the appeal letters, and we were denied there, too.

Ms. NORTON. Now, I am trying to establish whether or not in your cases we were dealing with specialists who recommended the treatment.

Ms. McCarty. Madam Chairman, my case, my oncologist recommended a bone marrow treatment for me. And I don't know how other patients went about investigating whether or not that was the right procedure for them, but I was very thorough, and I sought second opinions from Georgetown University and Lombardi Cancer Center, both which agreed. I obtained an opinion from Sloan–Kettering, which agreed. I obtained an opinion from Johns Hopkins, and they agreed. And I got an opinion from Georgetown—as I said, Georgetown, agreed.

So, in general, I think most patients do get second opinions. But, more specifically, no bone marrow transplant, I believe, in the United States, is ever administered without that being approved by the oncologist administering that bone marrow transplant.

Ms. Norton. And in the same way, did any of you deal directly with an insurance carrier who then said it is OPM's fault and not my fault? In other words, I am trying to establish whether the insurance carrier would have been willing to proceed had OPM been—not barred the payment for treatment.

Mr. Edward McKulsky. In my contacts with the Prudential Insurance Company of America, they told me because it wasn't part of my contract, they didn't have to cover it.

Ms. Norton. Of course, it is not a part of anybody's contract. So I am not sure what that means.

Mr. Edward McKulsky. It is just another way of saying that they weren't going to cover us because they didn't want to say experimental and investigational because their consultants hadn't seen all of our information yet.

Ms. Norton. For any of you, did the insurance carrier relate back to OPM or simply indicate its own policy?

Ms. Reger. Pardon me. I think that they indicated that their own policy didn't cover it. But I want you to understand that Blue Cross/Blue Shield tightened up their benefits in 1993. In 1993, they looked at these on a case-by-case basis, and if a reputable oncologist recommended it, maybe or maybe not they would fund it.

Ms. Norton. I mean in the Federal sector.

Ms. Reger. Under the Federal program. The health care benefits from Blue Cross/Blue Shield did not specifically exclude the treatment for breast cancer until 1993, and that is where I think they have gone amok. Because they do cover it for testicular cancer.

The preliminary trial data that was available in 1993 to make it appear as though it may not be the choice method, bone marrow transplant for testicular cancer. That is covered. Breast cancer is excluded. I am sure they are looking at the numbers of people and are afraid that everybody with breast cancer will want a bone marrow transplant. And, in fact, probably very few people with breast cancer will actually qualify for a bone marrow transplant. So I don't think we have to be so alarmed.

Ms. McCarty. Madam Chairman, May I add to that? If one is an astute shopper and trying to go about maneuvering your way through this maze of getting a bone marrow transplant, you don't generally enlist the help of OPM. So that the question that you are raising may not have really ever been addressed.

I looked at all the litigation against Blue Cross/Blue Shield with respect to the private sector, and I knew they had lost at least most, if not the majority, of their cases. So I tried to maneuver under the umbrella dealing with Blue Cross/Blue Shield directly. It was only when I had gotten my final denial from Blue Cross that they told me my redress at that time was to appeal to OPM. And after that point, I proceeded with OPM.

Ms. NORTON. The OPM role here, vis-a-vis the insurance carrier, is very troubling. OPM doesn't require it. If OPM doesn't require it, then we are left with whether or not any insurance company is going to do it, and to the possibility that the insurance company can use the fact that OPM doesn't require it enables them to simply deny it. And I am interested in what you said, Ms. Reger, about prior to 1993 in that regard.

Ms. REGER. That is right. I think if OPM requested a carrier who would cover bone marrow transplant for breast cancer, it would be in place. You have that coverage in Colorado, and they are going to have it, if not already, in Virginia. But as we are going State-by-State, getting victories with regard to some people getting this treatment, others are going to be dying because they don't have the time to wait.

Ms. MCCARTY. May I just add this to buttress your question? I went to visit the people administering this program at OPM. It was never clear to me whether or not OPM had the lead in requiring that this be a covered treatment or not. It was certainly my belief and I was led to believe that OPM did kind of act as the intermediary between the patient and the contract carrier. And it was also my opinion that, in speaking with OPM, they were predisposed to the belief that the treatment was experimental. And when Blue Cross/Blue Shield came back saying it was denied under their contract provisions, OPM just rubber-stamped that determination.

Ms. NORTON. Now, I am troubled here—I am not sure about—no one can know about your individual physicians or oncologists. But Ms. McCarty—it is Ms. McCarty—Ms. McCarty went to a world famous institution for treating cancer. And the Sloan institution hospital was—actually recommended this treatment or similar treatment for you?

Ms. MCCARTY. Yes.

Ms. NORTON. Now what I am trying to figure out is how NCI, OPM, or any insurance carrier, when they come up against an institution of that repute, can then say this is experimental and it—it is not proven enough to use. Could you tell me, therefore, what Sloan said to you when—when its agents recommended this treatment? Did Sloan say, "we are recommending this treatment to you, but it is not proven, and we don't think it will do much good." Were they more hopeful? What—on what basis, based on your conversations with the oncologists, did they recommend such a treatment to you at all if NCI says it is too experimental to be recommended?

Ms. MCCARTY. My conversation with the leading oncologist of the Breast Cancer Center there told me it has been their experience to date, under their protocol, that there their best success story was that there is a five-year survival rate. And they were very encouraging with respect to my entering their protocol. So that all I can say is that they were very encouraging. They thought it would be the best choice for me.

Ms. NORTON. It is very important for us to hear, given what we hear from OPM and even from the National Cancer Institute. Because we—one begins to wonder what is Sloan—what is Sloan doing? And I think Sloan is at least as reputable as the National Cancer Institute, if I may say so. So I am troubled by what you have testified to.

Let me ask all of you, the great feature of the FEHBP is said to be that we have these many carriers from which to choose, and you can shop around to find what may best suit your family, your own health needs, your own economic needs. Did any of you know before choosing your carrier that it would not cover this procedure or, for that matter, any procedures that would not be covered? And, if so, would you explain to us your experience?

Ms. REGER. Madam Chairman, there is no policy under OPM that covers bone marrow transplant for breast cancer. So you can shop all you want, but you are not going to find one. So those——

Ms. NORTON. My question is different. I know that. My question really has to do with whether or not you know in advance as you shop. No one can know if she is going to get breast cancer, but you know one in nine women do, and you know, therefore, if you think about it, you may not want a carrier that has limitations on breast cancer, assuming that you could find one. If you are a woman, that may be something that crosses your mind. And there may be other treatments that you want to know about.

And what I am trying to find out is how much information you have as to limitations with respect to available treatments.

Mr. EDWARD McKULSKY. Madam Chair, I think that most people, before they have a catastrophic illness in their family, when they look at these contracts that are handed out before the year, you are looking at cost. You are looking at benefits, general benefits. And I don't think people seriously look at the proper areas in these contracts.

One is what is excluded and general limitations. They should almost be put right in the front in bold print. Because if people realized what kind of coverage they had for catastrophic illnesses, I think it would help them make choices a lot better.

In our case, we had no choice because we didn't think we were going to have this problem. And as the one witness mentioned, I have seen over the last three years since we have been involved with this that the contracts have gotten stronger and more defined in wording to the point now that I believe they actually say that breast cancer is excluded.

Ms. McCARTY. Madam Chairman——

Ms. NORTON. My concern is, what kind of intermediary is OPM? You are absolutely right. If you had to sit down and read every contract, then you are in trouble. So if you have OPM there in the first place, one of the things this committee wants to know is if there is some kind of pass-through. Do they offer any service? Do they take into account precisely what you said?

There is nobody in the world that could sit down and read all these contracts, and yet some of these matters go to how OPM sells its service. It says look at all these things we give you. If it says look at all these things we give you, then it seems to me that there is some responsibility to pick out some items that are of increasing concern to the Federal employees who buy the polices. That is why I am trying to see if there is anything at the very least that the committee could recommend or require that OPM do so that people wouldn't end up shopping around, miss something that is important for them to know, or indeed why OPM doesn't have a carrier that might be willing to offer HDC treatment?

Ms. ROGERS. Madam Chairman, my experience is a little bit unique because I am not under the FEHBP program. The RTC/FDIC got a particular program of Blue Cross/Blue Shield. But, as I related in my testimony, they don't want to send you the contract because it is too large. Then OPM's not really doing their part, you know.

We finally requested, and once OPM and Blue Cross/Blue Shield knew we had filed a lawsuit, they said, well, you are going to have to file a formal request to get this contract. They didn't help us out in the procedures as we went along.

As I said, I read my benefits booklet very carefully. And I think it behooves the Office of Personnel Management to very clearly indicate these days what they do and do not cover. And if something changes, either additions or deletions, then those need to be communicated in a very timely fashion to all the employees that are under that particular plan.

Ms. MCCARTY. Madam Chairman, I would like to add to that with respect to your shopping issue. Generally, when you have a catastrophic illness of this nature, you are in the eye of a tornado. You don't even know what your next treatment option might be for your illness. So when the doctor told me that I needed a bone marrow transplant, I never even knew—I had no idea what that was. I mean, I didn't even know that it was within the spectrum of options of treatment for me. So, I could not make an informed shopping choice, because by the time I realized that I needed it, I was already in an existing plan. I had two months with which to take action.

Now, when I find out a woman has breast cancer that is employed by the Federal government, I tell her, in the future you may need a bone marrow transplant. When you select your health care plan with the Federal government, make sure that you select one that will cover that treatment.

So that goes to the second point which is that women don't know what they may need. And that is why in my testimony, I make the statement that in all these plans that don't cover it, there should be on the front a statement in bold language: This plan does not cover bone marrow transplants, and this is proven to be effective procedure for advanced cancer, for breast cancer. That way, women are put on notice there is something they should be aware of. You just don't know that information when you are told.

Ms. REGER. Madam Chair.

Ms. NORTON. Yes.

Ms. REGER. I am not even certain with a preexisting condition—you are a Federal employee. You want out of OPM because it is useless. I don't know that there is an insurer out there who would take you.

Ms. NORTON. And you certainly shouldn't have to get out of FEHBP altogether.

Ms. REGER. I had never seen it.

Ms. NORTON. Again, I recognize in part we are dealing with bureaucratic problems, what kind of information should be made available and what kind of information should not, and that we are dealing with, you know, tens and dozens and dozens of diseases and the rest.

Nevertheless, given the controversy that has arisen about this treatment—and I couldn't agree more with Ms. McCarty that, of course, in the eye of the tornado, you don't have a lot of basis for maneuverability. But the fact is that before the tornado, if what you are being sold is a menu of many plans, at least some generic information informing people of what is or is not available for example, if there was something that said—if there was information, let's say not on breast cancer but said to people so that it was understood that if a matter is in clinical trials, even if it shows promise, OPM does not recommend the two carriers that they are using.

The point here is that this controversy shows, above all, that almost everybody has been caught entirely unaware and have been left to compare themselves to others outside of the Federal system who have gotten easier access to this treatment.

And OPM need not think that it is protecting its carriers entirely from liability. Despite the fact that liability has not been found against one of its carriers yet, as this treatment improves, as these figures, these statistics show more promise, a carrier is not going to have OPM to hide behind. And given the kind of information that we are increasingly receiving, I would not like to be the lawyer for one of these carriers that is routinely denying this treatment. I think almost $90 million that one carrier has had to pay ought to be all the warning that is needed.

Mr. MYERS. Go to a jury trial.

Ms. NORTON. And you would get a jury trial and probably get a verdict.

Mrs. Morella, do you have any questions for these witnesses?

Mrs. MORELLA. No, I don't.

But, again, I want to thank the panel for testifying. I have learned a great deal from your personal experiences. I also learned that Virginia has a law, that medicaid pays for it. Boy, the evidence is all accumulating. Thank you very much.

Ms. NORTON. Mr. Myers.

Mr. MYERS. No, thank you. I talked to one witness about Tamoxifan. Thank you.

Ms. NORTON. Your testimony has been very helpful. We very much appreciate you coming forward.

Mrs. CATHARINE MCKULSKY. Thank you, Madam Chairman.

Ms. NORTON. Could we ask the next panel—Dr. Bruce Cheson, Head of the Medical Section, Clinical Investigations Branch, Division of Cancer Treatment, National Cancer Institute; Mr. Curtis Smith, Associate Director for Retirement Insurance, Office of Personnel Management.

STATEMENTS OF DR. BRUCE CHESON, HEAD, MEDICINE SECTION, CLINICAL INVESTIGATIONS BRANCH, DIVISION OF CANCER TREATMENT, NATIONAL CANCER INSTITUTE; AND CURTIS J. SMITH, ASSOCIATE DIRECTOR FOR RETIREMENT AND INSURANCE, OFFICE OF PERSONNEL MANAGEMENT

Mr. MYERS. If I might be recognized, Madam Chair.

Ms. NORTON. Yes, Mr. Myers.

Mr. MYERS. Curtis Smith, this is your last week. You are going to move over as the Federal executive in Charlottesville?

Mr. SMITH. Yes.

Mr. MYERS. Congratulations.

Mr. SMITH. Thank you very much.

Ms. NORTON. Put you in the firing line.

Mr. MYERS. He is expendable.

Ms. NORTON. Going to take the last shot.

Mr. SMITH. I will start, Doctor, if it is all right with you.

Good morning. Thank you for the opportunity to discuss the status of coverage under HDC/FEHBP for autologous bone marrow transplant with breast cancer.

With the Chair's permission, I will submit my statement——

Ms. NORTON. So ordered.

Mr. SMITH [continuing]. And summarize quickly.

We share the concerns that FEHBP needs to provide reasonable access to medically necessary treatments that have been demonstrated to be effective and all plans provide benefits for the treatment of cancer, including breast cancer. However, not all methods of treatment are covered under all plans, which is the issue we have before us today.

With ABMT—simply stated, the reason ABMT is not generally covered for treating certain conditions, such as breast cancer, is that in such cases, this treatment is not proven to be more effective than conventional treatments, while we know it carries a much higher risk. For this reason, OPM has not required carriers to cover the procedure, require that they carry the coverage.

Also, to aid in determining whether ABMT therapy for breast cancer is efficacious, OPM has arranged to allow FEHBP plans to participate in an outside non-FEHBP demonstration project sponsored by the Blue Cross and Blue Shield and the National Cancer Institute involving clinical trials in order to establish if both the trials are good and safe.

This issue is of serious concern to us at OPM, to FEHBP carriers, and certainly to our employees and their families. We will continue to actively monitor and review current published studies in the medical literature and to correspond with NCI and our FEHB's medical directors to update our knowledge of the HDC autologous bone marrow transplant for breast cancer while we await the results of the ongoing clinical trials.

We will not hesitate to modify FEHBP coverage requirements as soon as reliable clinical evidence indicates ABMT is as effective and worth the greater risk. We expressly advised our carriers in 1994 that once the clinical evidence establishes the efficacy and safety of ABMT for breast cancer, we would expect all plans to provide coverage, including changing coverage provisions in midyear.

And I will be happy to answer any questions you may have.

Ms. NORTON. Thank you very much.
[The prepared statement of Mr. Smith follows:]

PREPARED STATEMENT OF CURTIS J. SMITH, ASSOCIATE DIRECTOR FOR RETIREMENT
AND INSURANCE, OFFICE OF PERSONNEL MANAGEMENT

Madam Chair and Members of the Subcommittee: Thank you for this opportunity to discuss the status of coverage under the Federal Employees Health Benefits (FEHB) Program for autologous bone marrow transplants (ABMT) to support high dose chemotherapy in the treatment of breast cancer. Certainly, we share your concerns that the FEHB Program should provide reasonable access to medically necessary treatments that have been demonstrated to be effective.

The use of high doses of chemotherapy (HDC) to treat certain types of cancer is limited by the toxic effects on the patient's bone marrow cells and immune system. To counteract this, ABMT procedures involve removing bone marrow with its blood cell-producing agents from a patient before starting HDC and afterwards infusing that back into the patient to restore the immune system. This process involves great risk to the patient. Yet, ABMT has been widely accepted by the medical community for many years as effective in treating certain types of blood cancers, such as leukemias, and health insurance plans generally cover the therapy in such cases. Increasingly, patients with advanced breast cancer have sought this treatment as a last resort when other treatments have failed.

Over the past decade, use of ABMT to treat primary and advanced breast cancer has been the subject of ongoing clinical research. All of the expert medical opinion and published outcomes concerning this treatment that OPM has reviewed to date indicate that there is as yet no consensus in the medical community that ABMT in the treatment of breast cancer has proven to be as or more effective than conventional treatment. There is, however, widespread agreement that due to the toxicity, cost, and especially the complexity, evaluation of this treatment in randomized, comparative trials in major academic centers of excellence is warranted to document its effectiveness for breast cancer before it can be considered as part of the mainstream of conventional medicine. We maintain close contact with the National Cancer Institute (NCI) and they emphatically advise that ABMT therapy for breast cancer should not be performed outside of the clinical trial setting.

As administration of the FEHB Program, OPM does not generally mandate specific health plan coverages for particular diseases or conditions. The FEHB law specifies that broad types of medical services all plans should cover and plans basically provide benefits for such services whenever a qualified health care professional determines it is medically necessary. However, FEHB contracts state that the plan is not required to cover any treatments that are experimental or investigational, not medically necessary, or not rendered in accordance with generally accepted medical standards. The insurer, not OPM, determines the applicability of these general exclusions. OPM does not have the expertise, nor would it be appropriate, to make independent determinations as to the reasonableness, medical necessity, or efficacy of medical procedures. Nevertheless, when a benefit is not specifically excluded by the contract OPM may order a carrier to provide benefits in individual disputed claim class when our review of the specific evidence provided to us leads us to conclusions different from those of the carrier regarding the claimant's contractual entitlement to benefits.

Our policy is to require FEHB carriers to cover a procedure once it has become well-established in the medical community and the majority of insurers provide such coverage. This is not a determination by OPM regarding the medical status of the treatment or procedure, but rather a recognition of such determination by other competent authority and in attempt to conform the benefit structures of all competing FEHB plans so that consumers are not faced with surprises.

Accordingly, with respect to ABMT for breast cancer, OPM has not made any specific program-wide decision to cover or exclude treatment. Our position with respect to coverage for ABMT is based on its general acceptance in the medical community for each particular diagnosis.

All plans participating in the FEHB Program benefits for the treatment of cancer, including breast cancer. However, not all methods of treatment are covered under all plans. Simply stated, the reason ABMT is not generally covered for treating certain conditions, such as breast cancer, is that in such cases this treatment has not been proven to be more effective than conventional treatment, while we know it carries a much higher risk.

ABMT technology has been in use for many years, so it is not an experimental procedure. But the continuing clinical trials of ABMT in the treatment of breast cancer serve to define this mode of treatment as investigational for that condition and subject to general exclusion under FEHB contracts. While approximately 50 HMO-type FEHB plans currently provide coverage of this mode of treatment as a contract benefit, when determined by plan doctors to be medically necessary and appropriate, OPM does not require our plans to cover an investigative treatment.

Beginning with contract negotiations for 1993, though, we advised all plans that if they do not cover ABMT therapy for any condition, they must explicitly state this exclusion in plain language in the plan's benefit brochure to avoid any enrollee confusion and potential for litigation. The majority of FEHB plans, including the Blue Cross and Blue Shield Governmentwide Service Benefit Plan, at present exclude coverage of ABMT therapy for breast cancer.

Uniform FEHB coverage of ABMT for breast cancer is awaiting general acceptance by the medical community. Neither treatment costs nor popular sympathy are relevant factors in this decision; its a matter of assuring that the treatments help more than they harm. This is precisely the issue that ongoing clinical trials of these treatments are addressing.

However, in part to respond to increasing demands from FEHB enrollees and also to aid in determining whether ABMT therapy for breast cancer is efficacious, OPM has arranged to allow FEHB plans to participate in an outside, non-FEHB demonstration project sponsored by the Blue Cross and Blue Shield (BCBS) Association and the National Cancer Institute (NCI) involving clinical trials. In phase I of this project during 1991, only FEHB enrollees in the governmentwide service benefit plan could participate. We began phase II during 1992 when enrollees in other FEHB plans were eligible to participate. Presently, six fee-for-service plans and two HMOs have agreed to participate in and support these trials. We hope this expanded access to the clinical trials will hasten resolution of this important issue.

Medical facilities across the country are involved in the NCI ABMT trials. The trials accept qualified applicants at participating medical centers to be randomized into a regimen of conventional breast cancer treatment or treatment that uses ABMT. These trials are examining several different NCI-approved protocols and we hope they will provide a conclusive assessment of ABMT for the treatment of breast cancer. Blue Cross and Blue Shield handles the administrative arrangements for the demonstration project, including contracting with hospitals for discounted fees and processing applications from all potential enrollees, including FEHBP participants. Funding for the trials is provided by surcharges levied on participating private insurers; in the case of FEHB, OPM reimburses plans for the costs for each enrollee who is accepted and for the administrative costs that BCBS incurs. I wish to note, however, that although FEHBP funding is involved, OPM is not involved in administering the trials and we cannot require NCI to accept an enrollee into the trials if she does not meet the NCI protocols.

This is an issue of serious concern to OPM, FEHB carriers, and FEHB enrollees and their families. OPM will continue to actively monitor and review current published studies in the medical literature and to correspond with NCI and our FEHB plans' medical directors to update our knowledge of the status of HDC/ABMT therapy for breast cancer, while we await the results of the ongoing clinical trials. We will not hesitate to modify FEHB coverage requirements as soon as reliable clinical evidence indicates that ABMT is as effective for this condition as conventional treatment and is worth the greater patient risk. OPM expressly advised our carriers in the 1994 annual call letter for benefit and rate proposals that once clinical evidence establishes the efficacy and safety of ABMT for the treatment of breast cancer, we will expect all FEHB plans to provide coverage, including changing coverage provisions in mid-year.

I will gladly answer any questions you may have.

Ms. NORTON. Dr. Cheson.

Dr. CHESON. Yes. Thank you for the privilege of appearing before you today to discuss the status of the National Cancer Institute's position on autologous bone marrow transplantation as a treatment for breast cancer.

The National Cancer Institute is a biomedical research institution committed to generating the knowledge needed to reduce the suffering and death from cancer. At times, there have been bursts of enthusiasm for research advances that promised to cure cancer. However, we recognize that many patients with cancer still cannot be cured.

Today, there are exciting scientific developments on many fronts, particularly in basic research, but as we acknowledge these achievements, we must recognize that curing cancer poses an awesome challenge.

As you have already stated, cancer is the second leading cause of death among women in the United States. In 1994, about 250,000 women will die of all cancers combined, and of that number, about 46,000 will die from breast cancer. And breast cancer is the most common cause of death in women age 40 to 44. From 1973 until 1987, the incidence of breast cancer showed a steady increase. Therefore, this situation is critical.

I would like to turn to the procedure under discussion today, allogeneic bone marrow transplant or autologous bone marrow transplant. There are two procedures referred to as bone marrow transplants. The first type is autologous bone marrow transplantation in which the bone marrow is removed or harvested from a healthy donor and infused into a patient with a disease generally affecting the bone marrow. This procedure is effective for the treatments of diseases such as aplastic anemia and various forms of leukemia.

In the second type of procedure, an autologous transplant, the progenitor cells, or stem cells, are harvested either from the bone marrow or the peripheral blood of the patient with cancer. The patient is then treated with extremely high doses of chemotherapy, with or without radiation therapy.

Data from the laboratory in the clinic suggests that there is an increase in the responsiveness of tumors to chemotherapy when the dose of chemotherapy is increased, the so-called dose-response effect. Unfortunately, the dose we can deliver to a patient is often limited by the suppressive effects of these drugs on the patient's bone marrow.

The use of the patient's bone marrow as a form of rescue permits physicians to administer doses of drugs which are several times higher than can otherwise be tolerated. Without such support, the patient would be at great risk for lifethreatening or fatal complications of the therapy, particularly infections and bleeding.

Autologous bone marrow transplantation has been in clinical use for over a decade for patients with leukemias and other disorders of the blood and lymphatic system. More recently, it has been used to treat patients with solid tumors, such as breast cancer.

Data from the International Bone Marrow Transplant Registry show that the number of procedures performed in the United States for women with breast cancer has progressively increased from 265 in 1989 to more than 1,000 in 1993, such that it is now the most common form of cancer treated with this approach.

The initial studies of autologous bone marrow transplantation were performed in patients with advanced cancer who had failed more standard forms of treatment. Although response rates were very high, these responses lasted from only a few weeks to a few months and did not prolong survival. Moreover, 20 to 40 percent of patients died as a direct consequence of the procedure.

However, results from ABMT have improved considerably in recent years. Advances in supportive care using antibiotics and new drugs which stimulate a rapid return of the bone marrow have markedly reduced the complications and treatment-related deaths.

The increased experience of the physicians and their support staff have also contributed to the safe conduct of this procedure. Importantly, careful selection of patients most likely to benefit from this therapy has resulted in an improvement in the outcome.

Preliminary ABMT studies from individual, high-caliber institutions supported by the NCI such as Duke, the Dana-Farber Cancer Institute in Boston, the University of Colorado and the Anderson Cancer Center and others have provided encouraging results for the efficacy of ABMT for the treatment of women whose breast cancer has either spread to sites other than the breast, metastatic disease, or who are at high risk of recurring following their initial surgery.

Approximately 20 to 30 percent in these particular studies whose metastatic disease can be eradicated with standard chemotherapy may remain free of disease if they are also treated with autologous bone marrow transplantation. For women in the high-risk group, approximately 70 percent may experience a prolonged disease-free period with an excellent quality of life.

Whereas these results are encouraging, they must be viewed with care. First, they are often compared to treatments which would not be considered optimal today. We need to remember that continuing improvements in our standard treatments have enabled us to cure an increasing number of women, particularly in the high-risk group.

Second, the published transplant experience includes highly selected women who are otherwise in good health, who are highly motivated and who have other features which predict that they will respond to and tolerate this therapy well.

In addition, published information is generated from investigators who are extremely qualified to perform this toxic therapy. Therefore, we are faced with one of the most important and certainly one of the most controversial and unanswered questions in cancer therapy: Is autologous bone marrow transplantation better than current standard therapy in comparable breast cancer patients?

To address this important question, the NCI is sponsoring three national, high-priority multi-institutional clinical trials, two for women at high risk of recurrence and one for women with metastatic disease. To date, more than 1,000 women have entered onto these studies at more than 70 institutions around the country. Each study is halfway to a completion of its accrual.

The fact that these studies will take several more years to be completed and analyzed does not mean that research in this field is being delayed. While these definitive comparative trials are ongoing, developmental studies are being conducted at various cancer centers to improve on the treatment of breast cancer, including the use of ABMT.

Therefore, while this treatment is promising, there are a number of concerns that need to be addressed before it can be considered standard therapy.

First, we need to be able to identify patients who are most likely to benefit so that the others can receive more appropriate treatment. For example, ABMT should not be considered as a treatment of last resort, for it is in those patients for whom it is least likely to be of benefit.

Second, we are dealing with a very expensive form of therapy which must be used appropriately because of its cost. Efforts made by some investigators have demonstrated that it is possible to significantly reduce the cost without compromising patient safety.

Third, this therapy is being increasingly delivered by inexperienced physicians outside of clinical trials who are less familiar with dealing with the life-threatening complications of the treatment which jeopardizes patient safety and reduces the likelihood of benefit.

Last, we are not satisfied with the current results of this treatment and recognize the need to improve on its efficacy in breast cancer as well as other diseases.

The NCI believes that clinical trials of ABMT for the treatment of patients with tumors such as breast cancer are essential to determine the safety and efficacy of this procedure. Only through the conduct of well-designed prospective studies can we determine if this approach is of benefit, including the specific diseases and patient groups for which it is appropriate.

Currently, NCI-sponsored clinical trials are carefully addressing these important issues. For patients with breast cancer, more data are needed to definitively establish the roll of ABMT as standard therapy. Although it is not within the mandate of the NCI to determine coverage policy, we believe it is scientifically and clinically responsible for formal scientific evaluation to precede the routine use of such a toxic and expensive therapy in clinical practice. We believe routine use in clinical practice should occur only after scientific evaluation establishes its value. In the case of ABMT, this has not yet definitively occurred.

Currently, ABMT is also being evaluated in certain patients with leukemias, lymphomas, multiple myeloma, testicular cancer, ovarian cancer and some childhood malignancies. We have made considerable progress; however, for such advances to continue, we need continued support of the clinical trials process.

The NCI affirms its commitment to reduce death and suffering from breast cancer, and this commitment is made with a full awareness of its awesome challenge. Through basic research and clinical trials in both prevention and treatment, we believe we have made progress and will continue to make progress in the continuing battle against breast cancer.

Thank you for this opportunity to testify, and I would be pleased to answer any questions.

Ms. NORTON. Thank you very much, Dr. Cheson.

[The prepared statement of Dr. Cheson follows:]

PREPARED STATEMENT OF DR. BRUCE CHESON, HEAD, MEDICINE SECTION, CLINICAL INVESTIGATIONS BRANCH, DIVISION OF CANCER TREATMENT, NATIONAL CANCER INSTITUTE

Madam Chairwoman, and Members of the Subcommittee, I am Dr. Bruce Cheson, Head of the Medicine Section, Clinical Investigations Branch, Division of Cancer Treatment, National Cancer Institute. Thank you for the privilege of appearing before you today to discuss the National Cancer Institute's position on autologous bone marrow transportation as a treatment for breast cancer.

The National Cancer Institute (NCI) is a biomedical research institution committed to generating the knowledge needed to reduce the suffering and death from caner. At times there have been bursts of enthusiasm for research advances that promised to cure cancer; however we all recognize that many patients with cancer still cannot be cured. Today, there are exciting developments on many fronts, particularly in basic research, but as we acknowledge these achievements, we must recognize that cancer poses an awesome research and therapeutic challenge.

What is clear is that the practice of cancer therapy will require adjustments or fundamental changes as we learn more about the biology and immunology of cancer cells, and have more opportunity to assess diagnostic tools and treatments. We have seen that yesterday's "incurable and fatal" disease can be tomorrow's medical triumph, and that a disease that terrorizes one generation may be only dimly remembered by the next generation. In light of this, two principles need to guide us whenever possible: the review of research by scientific peer groups, and clinical trials as the instrument for the development of new treatments.

Cancer is the second leading cause of death among women in the United States. In 1994, about 250,000 women will die of all cancers combined; of that number about 46,000 will die from breast cancer. Breast cancer is the most common cause of death from any cause in women aged 40–44. From 1973 until 1987 the incidence of breast cancer showed a steady increase. Since 1987, breast cancer incidence, fortunately, has reached a plateau and has actually decreased slightly. Nevertheless, the situation is critical.

Turning to the procedure under discussion today, autologous bone marrow transplantation (ABMT) as a treatment for breast cancer. There are two procedures which are generally referred to as bone marrow transplants. The first type is allogeniec bone marrow transplantation, in which bone marrow is removed, or harvested, from a healthy donor and infused into a patient with a disease generally affecting the bone marrow or immune system. This procedure is effective for the treatment of diseases such as aplastic anemia and various forms of leukemia. In the second type of procedure, an autologous transplant, the progenitor cells, or stem cells, are harvested from either the bone marrow or peripheral blood of a patient with cancer. The patient is then treated with extremely high doses of chemotherapy with or without radiation therapy. Because this treatment is capable of eradicating the patient's own bone marrow, the harvested stem cells are then administered back into the patient to hasten the recovery of the patient's own bone marrow function. Without such support, the patient would be at great risk for life threatening or fatal complications of the chemotherapy, particularly infections and bleeding.

Autologous bone marrow transplantation has been in clinical use for over a decade for patients with leukemias and other disorders of the blood and lymphatic system. More recently it has been used to treat patients with solid tumors, such as breast caner. Data from the International Bone Marrow Transplant Registry show that the number of procedures performed in the U.S. for women with breast cancer has progressively increased from 265 in 1989, to more than 1,000 in 1993, such that it is now the most common form of cancer treated with this approach.

Data from the laboratory and from clinical trials sponsored by NCI and other research organizations suggest that there is an increase in the responsiveness of tumors to chemotherapy with an increase in the administered doses, a so-called dose-response effect. Unfortunately, the dose we can deliver to a patient is often limited by the suppressive effects of these drugs on the patient's bone marrow. The use of a patient's bone marrow as a form of rescue permits physicians to administer doses of drugs which are several times higher than can otherwise be tolerated.

The initial studies of autologous bone marrow transplantation were conducted in patients with advanced cancer who had failed more standard forms of treatment. Although response rates were very high, these responses lasted from a few weeks to several months, and did not prolong survival. Moreover, 20–40 percent of patients died as a direct consequence of the procedure. However, results from autologous transplantation have improved considerably in recent years. Advances in supportive care using antibiotics and new drugs which stimulate a rapid return of the bone marrow have markedly reduced the complications and treatment-related deaths. The increased experience of the physicians and their support staff have also contributed to the safe conduct of this procedure. Importantly, careful selection of patients most likely to benefit from this therapy has resulted in an improvement in the outcome. These outcomes are first seen through clinical trials research.

Clinical trials research is important in developing new approaches to cancer treatment and prevention. Breast cancer clinical trials have led to the availability of improved diagnostic tests, have proven the value of less extensive surgery, have refined techniques used in breast reconstruction, and have increased survival. NCI supports a large network of Community Clinical Oncology Programs (CCOPs), Cooperative Groups, and Cancer Centers that provide state-of-the-art care for patients and perform clinical trials designed to develop better therapies. In 1971, NCI supported three comprehensive cancer centers; today we support 28 such centers across the country, together with 30 other specialized centers that receive grant support. The comprehensive cancer centers have a mandate to bring advances in cancer prevention, detection, and treatment to their communities and to develop strong links with community physicians and support groups. The Clinical Cooperative Groups Program began in 1975 and initially conducted small studies with few patients. The Groups now conduct approximately 35 breast cancer treatment trials that enroll approximately 5,000 new patients each year. The establishment of CCOPs in 1983 created a network of community cancer specialist, primary care physicians, and other health care professionals who conduct research on clinical treatment, cancer prevention and control, screening, chemoprevention, smoking cessation, patient management, continuing care, and rehabilitation. The program involves more than 300 hospitals and nearly 2,500 physicians.

Preliminary ABMT studies from individual, high caliber institutions supported by NCI such as Duke University, the Dana Farber Cancer Institute in Boston, the University of Colorado, and others, have provided encouraging results for the efficacy of ABMT treatment in women whose breast cancer has either spread to sites other than the breast (metastatic cancer), or who are at a high risk of recurring following their initial surgery. Approximately 20–30 percent of women in these particular studies whose metastic disease can be eradicated with standard chemotherapy may remain free of disease if they are also treated with ABMT. For women in the high risk group, approximately 70% may experience a prolonged disease free period with an excellent quality of life.

Whereas these results are encouraging, they must be viewed with care. First of all, they are often compared to treatments which would not be considered optimal today. We need to remember that continuing improvements in our standard treatments have enabled us to cure an increasing number of women, particularly in the high risk group. Second, the transplant series includes a very highly selective group of women who are otherwise in good health, who are highly motivated, and who have other features which predict that they will respond to and tolerate this therapy well. In addition, the investigators who are involved are extremely qualified to perform this toxic therapy. Therefore, we are faced with one of the most important and certainly one of the most controversial and unanswered questions in cancer therapy: Is autologous bone marrow transplantation better than current standard therapy in comparable breast cancer patients?

To address this important question, NCI is sponsoring three national, high priority multi-institutional clinical trials; two for women at high risk of recurrence, and one for women with metastatic disease. To date, 1,000 women have entered into these studies at more than 70 institutions around the country, and each study is half-way to completion of accrual.

The fact that these studies will take several more years to be completed does not mean that research in this field is being delayed. While these definitive comparative trials are ongoing, developmental studies are being conducted at various cancer centers to improve on the treatment of breast cancer, including the use of autologous bone marrow transplantation.

Therefore, while this treatment is promising, there are a number of concerns that need to be addressed before it is considered "standard" therapy. First, we need to be able to identify patients who are the most likely to benefit so that the others can receive more appropriate treatment. For example, ABMT should not be considered a treatment of last resort, for it is in those patients for whom it is least likely to be of benefit. Second, we are dealing with a very expensive form of therapy which must be used appropriately because of its cost. Efforts made by some investigators, such as Dr. Williams Peters at Duke University, have demonstrated that it is possible to significantly reduce the cost without compromising patient safety. Third, this therapy is being increasingly delivered by inexperienced physicians outside of clinical trials who are less familiar with dealing with the life-threatening complications of this treatment, which jeopardizes patient safety and reduces the likelihood of benefit. Last, we are not satisfied with the current results of this form of treatment and recognize the need to improve on its efficacy in breast cancer as well as other diseases.

The NCI believes that clinical trials of ABMT for the treatment of patients with tumors such as breast cancer, are essential to determine the safety and efficacy of this procedure. Only through the conduct of well-designed prospective studies can we determine if this approach is of benefit, including the specific diseases and specific patient groups for which it is appropriate. Currently, NCI sponsored clinical trials are carefully addressing these important issues. For patients with breast cancer, more data are needed to definitively establish the role of ABMT as standard therapy in these disease settings. Although it is not within the mandate of the NCI to determine coverage policy, we believe it is scientifically and clinically responsible for formal scientific evaluation to precede the routine use of such a toxic and expensive therapy in clinical practice. We believe that routine use in clinical practice should occur only after scientific evaluation establishes its value. In the case of ABMT this has not yet occurred.

Currently, ABMT is also being evaluated in the treatment of certain patients with leukemias, lymphomas, multiple myeloma, testicular cancer, ovarian cancer, and some childhood malignancies. We have made considerable progress; however, for such advances to continue, we need continued support of the clinical trials process. Each of us has a role to play in this enormously important effort to save the lives of American women.

The NCI has an important mandate to inform the scientific community and the public regarding advances in our knowledge about cancer. The PDQ (Physician Data Query) system is available via several routes (including computer modem, CD–ROM, and fax) to physicians, other health care professionals, and the public. PDQ includes up-to-date information on state-of-the-art therapy and clinical trials supported by NCI. The public can obtain information about cancer from the NCI Cancer Information Service. A trained information specialist can be reached by calling the toll-free phone number 1–800–4–CANCER.

The NCI affirms its commitment to reduce death and suffering from breast cancer and this commitment is made with a full awareness of its awesome challenge. Through basic research and clinical trials in both prevention and treatment we believe we have made progress and will continue to make progress in the continuing battle against breast cancer.

Thank you for this opportunity to testify. I would be pleased to answer any questions you or other members of the subcommittee may have.

Ms. NORTON. Let me preface my questions, particularly to Dr. Cheson, by saying that I have a great respect for the way in which scientific evidence must be accrued. I particularly followed the way in which persons with AIDS have felt about pressing beyond trials. I understand perfectly what it takes and what it should take to prove the efficacy of a particular treatment. And myself, an academic, still teach a course at Georgetown Law School and have great respect for the kind of research it takes to prove anything, whether it is a matter in law or a matter of scientific evidence.

Let me ask you first, Dr. Cheson, has the Sloan institution ever taken part in your clinical trials?

Dr. CHESON. Memorial Sloan–Kettering does take part in our clinical trials. They also have other trials which they conduct independently through other resources.

Ms. NORTON. Yes. How would you characterize Sloan's reputation in the scientific community?

Dr. CHESON. Memorial Sloan–Kettering is considered one of the finest cancer centers in the country and was, in fact, rated number one in a recent poll that appeared in—I forget which one of the business magazines. It is an excellent institution.

Ms. NORTON. You wouldn't consider it malpractice for Sloan to recommend a treatment similar to the one under discussion here for a patient who comes to Sloan?

Dr. CHESON. It would depend on the patient. Different patients have different likelihoods of benefiting from this procedure.

Ms. NORTON. So that if a patient is likely to benefit from this procedure, Dr. Cheson, you believe that it is consistent with sound medical practice to allow the treatment?

Dr. CHESON. The National Cancer Institute's position is that the therapy would be appropriate if conducted in the clinical trial setting.

Ms. NORTON. Well, if an institution like Sloan ordered the treatment outside of a clinical trial setting, would you believe that Sloan was doing something inappropriate?

Dr. CHESON. It would be unlikely that they would do that, since they have a number of clinical trials for patients with this particular condition.

Ms. NORTON. So you believe that Sloan is only allowing this treatment in clinical trials?

Dr. CHESON. I can't speak for them, not knowing all the patients they have treated. But we recommend that patients only receive this therapy on clinical trials, not necessarily these large randomized trials which are taking years to complete. But there are developmental studies that are ongoing at cancer centers from which useful information will be learned so that we can improve on the results of this treatment. Institutions like Memorial Sloan–Kettering are conducting those sorts of studies, and they have a very fine program.

Ms. NORTON. So while you recommend that the treatment be administered only in clinical trials, I take it that is controlled studies?

Dr. CHESON. Not necessarily. Developmental studies are also ongoing using new forms of high-dose therapy and other methods intended on improving its efficacy and reducing the toxicities that aren't necessarily controlled trials which, if they appear to be an advance, are then taken to controlled trials.

But these need to be conducted at an institution with the ability to perform high-quality clinical trials so that the patient is not being subjected to the risks of this procedure without something at least being learned from it that can benefit that patient or at least future patients.

Ms. NORTON. So while the NCI recommends that this treatment be administered in clinical trials, you are not prepared to say it is inappropriate for it to be recommended outside of clinical trials?

Dr. CHESON. It would depend on the setting in which it is being conducted. If it is being conducted at an institution which is experienced in the conduct of clinical trials and has some form of quality assurance, institutional review, et cetera, that is fine.

But what I am saying is that there are now a large number of small hospitals that are undertaking this procedure which is being performed by individuals who lack the experience and expertise to do this safely and from which no useful information will be gained to improve this field and to improve on therapy.

Ms. NORTON. That is why the premise of all of my questions, Dr. Cheson, have been Sloan. I understand that we don't want Podunk hospital.

Dr. CHESON. But that is what is being done.

Ms. NORTON. That may be what is being done. But I am not talking about Podunk hospital. I am submitting to you an institution which you yourself say is the number one in the country.

And, indeed, we have testimony from an attorney, Robert Carter, that suggests that many of the country's top medical institutions refuse to participate in NCI trials because they believe that HDC/ABMT treatment is far superior to conventional treatment and that the continued use of randomized trials is, at least in this situation, unethical. Do you propose that conventional treatment is superior to the HDC treatment results obtained thus far?

Dr. CHESON. I would hope that the high-dose chemotherapy is superior. It remains to be demonstrated. And I would take issue with whoever makes comments that these randomized trials are unethical. I think that sort of statement is inappropriate.

Ms. NORTON. Does there come a point when our knowledge of a treatment is such that randomized trials would be unethical?

Dr. CHESON. Absolutely. Well, not unethical. Because, let's say under the best of circumstances, with the current status of this therapy, 70 percent of women experienced long-term, disease-free survival. That means that 30 percent are dying. There still needs to be improvement. But there comes a time when the therapy, as is currently being used, may be considered "standard." But that is the point we need to move from.

Ms. NORTON. What is that point? What is standard? Give me an example from your own experience of a treatment that has started as experimental and then it got to X point and you then considered that it was ready to be regarded as standard.

What is X point? Is it a percentage of women who live as opposed to patients who live against those who die? Or is there some other unit of evaluation that you use?

Dr. CHESON. I think a general unit evaluation would be that it is at least as good as and not significantly more toxic than the treatments that are available at that particular time.

Ms. NORTON. Now we are faced with the fact—and this would be a substantial concern to this committee—that a substantial number of court cases have specifically rejected the argument that this treatment for breast cancer is experimental.

Now, courts aren't doctors, but they listen to both sides. And there would be the concern in this committee if carriers, in following the NCI recommendation, were, in fact, submitting themselves to $90 million lawsuits, to take one example. How would you comment on these adverse decisions of courts? And have you taken that into account as you wait to somehow reach the level of standard care?

Dr. CHESON. We still believe that it is most appropriate to conduct this form of therapy in the context of peer review clinical trials. These trials are open from coast to coast in all of the United States and are open for the vast majority of women for whom this therapy would be considered to be appropriate.

I can't speak to all the details of the California case. It is my understanding there were some other issues concerning the insurance company itself and not primarily the procedure. But I am not familiar with all the details.

We do not like to use the word "experimental" or the word "investigational" because they are vague. They mean different things to different people. We prefer to base determinations on whether it is appropriate for a particular patient and whether, based on the appropriateness, it should be considered standard treatment.

Ms. NORTON. Now, of course, the OPM policy makes it inappropriate for any patient, as far as they are concerned, because they don't require it. And that says to the carriers who can't wait to find a way to save money, don't do it.

Dr. CHESON. There are many carriers who are now approving this therapy performed on appropriate patients on peer review clinical trials.

Ms. NORTON. But not for Federal employees.

Dr. CHESON. I can't speak to that, although I am a Federal employee.

Mr. SMITH. May I speak the that, Madam Chair?

Ms. NORTON. Yes, Mr. Smith—be glad to have you speak to that.

Mr. SMITH. Because it is really an important issue that you have raised. We do, in fact, provide access to our employees to the NCI clinical trials.

Ms. NORTON. I am aware of that, yes.

Mr. SMITH. But I think that what really is the issue here is that we have made a precedent here. We have never done this before where we paid the expenses for a procedure that wasn't yet a standard procedure. But this one seems so important that we set the precedent.

Ms. NORTON. Why did you make an exception here?

Mr. SMITH. Because it seems as important to us as it seems to you.

Ms. NORTON. Importance is a word that is completely vague to me. Everything is important if it involves somebody's life. Why did you decide that we are going to pay for clinical trials here, even though we have never done that before?

Mr. SMITH. Because of the number of people affected, the seriousness of the disease. I mean, we have heard the numbers this morning about what a really serious, widespread problem this is.

Ms. NORTON. It had nothing to do with the fact that the treatment has been found increasingly effective?

Mr. SMITH. Not at the time. We did not know that at the time this decision was made three or four years ago.

Ms. NORTON. My goodness, you mean to say you would have made that decision even if the scientific evidence was that it didn't do any good just because there were a lot of folk who were affected?

Mr. SMITH. We made the decision so that we could have the scientific evidence to answer this question and know whether or not we should make it a standard procedure.

Ms. NORTON. It had nothing to do with whether or not you were being affected by the promise that the trials are beginning to show?

Mr. SMITH. Maybe I am misunderstanding the question. If everyone had been writing off this procedure as useless, it is unlikely we would have done this, of course. Sure.

Ms. NORTON. I am trying to get on the record that you knew that you had not just a lot of women out here, not just a serious disease, but you were aware of the fact that you had a treatment that was increasingly promising.

Mr. SMITH. And that NCI was devoting a great deal of its efforts also to pursue.

Ms. NORTON. They are devoting a great deal of their efforts to a lot of treatments.

The reason I am asking this is that we are here to try to find out how OPM makes these decisions. And, therefore, it is important for us to know the basis for them or otherwise we are left to what we keep hearing; that you do it on the basis of sex discrimination or—so I want to know. Is one ingredient that, well, it looks like it is getting somewhere and, therefore, we ought to pay for the trials?

Mr. SMITH. Certainly.

Ms. NORTON. Thank you.

Go ahead. I am sorry. I didn't mean to stop you.

Mr. SMITH. No, no. I think I made the point that I wanted to, that the—and these are sort of national health issues, too. I don't know what all the answers need to be. But we have, as a program, for 30 years not wanted to require payment for things that were experimental or investigational. And saw——

Ms. NORTON. Dr. Cheson says you are wrong to even use that word. That you ought to be doing this on an "as appropriate", case-by-case basis.

Mr. SMITH. Well, okay. Then we have only paid for things that——

Mr. NORTON. This is your consultant.

Mr. SMITH [continuing]. That were standard, accepted practices, which I think is the meaning of the words that I was using.

The real issue here, I think, is that nobody that we have heard from is recommending that this procedure—I mean, the people at Duke and places like that, everybody is saying that procedures should be done in a clinical trial setting. And we have looked for a way and found initially the NCI approach to paying for the procedure in that context for people in FEHBP.

Ms. NORTON. Mr. Smith, you have got to help me out here. I asked this question earlier of people who didn't have your expertise and background. It really has to do with insurance carriers who are not out there trying to find treatments to pay for these days. And yet we find that non-Federal plans increasingly pay for this. Now, how are we, therefore, to interpret OPM's policy, when insurance carriers all over the country are indeed paying for this treatment?

Mr. SMITH. I can't tell you.

Ms. NORTON. Can you explain that?

Mr. SMITH. I can explain what we do. I can't explain, of course, what others are doing.

And what we have been doing here is to say that until it is standard practice, accepted as standard practice in the medical community, that we don't think that we should require carriers to cover it. We don't deny it when someone comes forward and wants to, for whatever reasons prompts them to do that. But we do not require it until it is accepted as standard practice.

Ms. NORTON. I have a number of other questions, but I want to catch Mrs. Morella before she leaves to ask if she has any questions.

Mrs. MORELLA. Thank you very much.

I want to thank you both for testifying. We have been looking forward to your testimony.

Dr. Cheson, you are at the NCI, the National Institutes of Health, and I am very proud of the work you have been doing there and have been very supportive. You know, these clinical trials, it is awfully tough to be a part of them, isn't it? Don't you have strict eligibility rules? Would you tell us what they are?

Dr. CHESON. Well, they vary with the particular clinical trial. And, no, they are not hard to get into.

For example, if you go to Duke—which we have heard mentioned numerous times—and other cancer centers, you cannot receive this therapy unless you are on a clinical trial. They will not administer it off a clinical trial setting.

Clinical trials will generally require that a patient be—the generic clinical trial—the patient have reasonably normal organ function, such as their kidneys work reasonably well, their heart works reasonably well and any other organ that might be damaged by the therapy that is being planned. In this case, their heart function should be adequate and their lung function.

Generally there is an upper age based on—not on chronology but on the patient's overall performance. There is generally an issue of what we call performance data, how that patient can function. A patient who is bedridden and moribund would not survive this procedure. There are basic physiologic guidelines we use.

Then there are certain situations in which we know that the therapy will not work. If a patient, for example, with breast cancer has failed multiple treatments for metastatic disease, we know that then giving them, based on data from Duke and elsewhere, giving them high dose therapy, while it may achieve a response, the response is extremely transient and may just be a matter of a few weeks to a couple of months and of very little benefit. In that particular setting, that is where we have these developmental trials which are using more, newer therapies, new approaches, new drugs.

So, to answer your question more directly, there are certain basic physiological guidelines that we use as well as those that we have learned based on our prior experience and treatment of those diseases.

Mrs. MORELLA. Is somebody exempt from consideration of a trial if that person has had chemotherapy before?

Dr. CHESON. It would depend on the study. If a woman had been given chemotherapy, they would not be exempt for a study at the time they recurred for a metastatic disease study.

We have, in fact, expanded our eligibility criteria for the three large national studies that I mentioned to try to make them much more user friendly, permitting more, prior therapy, broadening the eligibility criteria to keep them within safe limits but broadening them, expanding the number of institutions. So we have tried to be as flexible as possible without sacrificing safety and without sacrificing the scientific integrity of the study.

Mrs. MORELLA. But you know, obviously, there are going to be a lot of people who are not going to be allowed to become part of these trials because of the flip of the coin, the numbers you are going to have, the eligibility you say which you say you are beginning to relax and expand. And these may be the people—obviously, I believe would be the people who would probably benefit most by the results of being part of the trial.

You also mention you don't like the term "experimental" or whatever. But I think the term the insurance companies use is investigational, right?

Dr. CHESON. Right.

Mrs. MORELLA. What does that mean?

Dr. CHESON. Your guess is as good as mine.

Investigational generally is taken to mean something that has not yet been proven to be standard therapy, which runs the gamut from the first time you put a drug into a patient that has never been given to a patient before, all the way to an agent which has demonstrated efficacy but has not been to the point of "proven." That is why it is such a vague term.

There are a lot of therapies that looked promising but didn't pan out. We hope high-dose chemotherapy will turn out to be better, but we need to select the people who are going to benefit. Because there are a lot of people who get this who really have no chance of benefiting from it.

Mrs. MORELLA. Or it may be—excuse me. It may be what you said that you don't like to give it to those people where it is the last resort. But the mere fact that it is the last resort and does make a difference in terms of life, I would think would be an appealing feature of offering it.

If a doctor, expert, diagnoses someone and says, this is your chance to live. Otherwise, there is no hope. We think there is a very good chance, maybe a 60 percent chance, that you are going to be around for a long period of time. I just think that——

Dr. CHESON. When I said last resort, what I was referring to is somebody who failed multiple therapies, who is exceptionally ill, who is frail and fragile, and there is really nothing else that works. That is the sort of person who couldn't even tolerate this form of treatment, not the person who has been told, yes, you have breast cancer, and this is an appropriate treatment for you.

There is a difference in the definitions there. The therapy should be offered to appropriate patients at appropriate centers who are conducting clinical research.

Mrs. MORELLA. Is Georgetown an appropriate center?

Dr. CHESON. Absolutely. And they are participating in the NCI clinical trials.

Mrs. MORELLA. But they are also treating people who may not be part of the trial, right?

Dr. CHESON. They are also an NCI-funded comprehensive cancer center. Therefore, their clinical protocols on which they are treating these patients have undergone peer review. So although they are not part of these big trials, as I said before, we sponsor many developmental studies which are looking at improving this treatment. Because for certain groups of patients, it is really not very good.

Mrs. MORELLA. That is fascinating. That is exactly what I wanted to hear.

Ms. NORTON. Would the gentlelady yield on that for one second?

This is to Mr. Smith. The protocols that have been approved, as Dr. Cheson just said, at Georgetown, the respect that clearly he indicates the institution is held, still does not warrant your approval, OPM's approval, of NCI treatment programs as opposed to NCI trials, which you in fact do fund?

Mr. SMITH. That is correct. The step we have taken is with the NCI trials, the three large ones that Dr. Cheson has spoken of.

Mrs. MORELLA. You can see the benefit of this treatment when you consider that, as you said, ages 40 to 44, the highest mortality.

So when you think of these people as mothers, wives, daughters and what it can mean to themselves and their families, it indicates how important this period is and how important these trials are. And I have an impatience in terms of how long it is going to take before we take it out of that investigational category and say this is a treatment to be used.

Dr. CHESON. I should mention that all these trials are being conducted, the data are analyzed at regular intervals by independent scientists who are not—have no vested interest in whether it works or not. So there is no conflict of interest. And if, at some time along the conduct of this trial, there is sufficient reason to believe that the therapies are significantly different, then the studies will be terminated early. So if we find out that it is better, we are not going to continue plugging on just for the sake of plugging on.

Mrs. MORELLA. And, Mr. Smith, you say that OPM will accept it, but they don't suggest it. They don't require it. So it is kind of a chilling effect, in a way, for anybody, any company saying, yes, we will pay for it. What is the percentage? Are there any of the providers that do offer it now under the FEHB program?

Mr. SMITH. Out of the NCI trial arrangement, no, very few people cover it. There are a number of HMOs throughout the country on the fee-for-service side. None of the open fee-for-service nationwide plans cover it outside—some of those larger plans do participate in the NCI clinical trials. But, no, there is not very much coverage. You are right about that.

Ms. NORTON. Would the gentlewoman yield?

In fact, OPM covers treatment for these HMOs, as well, does it not? You just mentioned HMOs as also covering treatment. I mean, but you pay HMOs that cover this treatment?

Mr. SMITH. Yes. And I should make a distinction, too, between the relationship in FEHBP between the fee-for-service plans on one hand and the HMOs on the other.

With the HMOs, we buy the community package at the community rate and don't have the kind of discussions about benefits and costs, for example, that we have with the fee-for-service plans. So what you will see in the HMO world is that whatever the HMOs do in that community is what we are asking them to provide for Federal employees.

Mrs. MORELLA. How does OPM respond to State laws? Are you exempt from them because it is Federal?

Let's say—I understand Virginia, I heard today, has a law that would require private providers to cover this treatment. How does OPM look to the States for their laws and insurance commissions?

Mr. SMITH. You are right. Our statute exempts us from State laws that make our plans inconsistent from State to State. I understand and we have heard a couple of times this morning concerns about the fact that in a particular State Federal employees may be treated differently than other citizens of that State. Our overriding concern has been that our people be treated sort of consistently across the Nation, and that is really where the exemption comes from.

Most large employers with self-insured plans are exempt from State mandates in order to provide a consistent policy across all the States to a large work force.

Mrs. MORELLA. Well, I guess Maryland doesn't have that law that Virginia has. I am going to have to talk to some State legislators maybe in the gubernatorial campaign. We will get something moving in that regard.

Mr. SMITH. The oldest use of ABMT has been for things like leukemia, and other uses have been relatively recent, in, I would say, the last couple of years.

Mrs. MORELLA. You accepted it for the FEHBP coverage a couple years ago?

Mr. SMITH. Yes. So plans cover it. I don't know right now if everybody does.

Mrs. MORELLA. Are they through the clinical trials and evaluation?

Dr. CHESON. The problem with testicular cancer is it is such an uncommon tumor that to conduct a randomized trial would take absolutely forever. And, as a result, you are much more reliant on historical data.

Mrs. MORELLA. There is——

Dr. CHESON. Therein is a problem.

Mrs. MORELLA. There is a gap right there.

Ms. NORTON. Would the gentlewoman yield?

Dr. CHESON. It is not black and white.

Ms. NORTON. Without the kind of clinical evidence that you require, because it would take too long to get, you said go ahead and do the treatment?

Dr. CHESON. Unless things are much more clearly black and white. If, for example, a patient receiving third-line therapy for testicular cancer, 100 percent die within six months, and you do this procedure and 50 percent are alive, then you really don't need very much.

If things are in the gray zone, as they are with breast cancer where patients treated with standard therapy, in fact, do survive a long time, whether it is as many as with high-dose therapy is what is not clear. Then you have a problem, and that is where you have to determine whether therapies are comparable or not, particularly when one is so much more toxic and so expensive than the other.

Mrs. MORELLA. Just one final point. You ever get involved in litigation—I mean, as a witness?

Dr. CHESON. Do I?

Mrs. MORELLA. In cases like this. Yes. Do you ever get called into court?

Dr. CHESON. As a representative of the National Cancer Institute, we are not allowed to.

Mrs. MORELLA. I was going to say for your expert opinion.

Dr. CHESON. As a private citizen, I am frequently asked my expert opinion.

Mrs. MORELLA. Thank you very much. I think you both know where I am coming from and I think the subcommittee is coming from. Thank you.

Ms. NORTON. Thank you, Miss Morella.

Mr. Myers.

Mr. MYERS. Thank you, Madam Chair.

I have learned something this morning from all the witnesses. First, my experience with cancer that ABMT was a last resort. Now, I am hearing this morning it is primary therapy in some cases if the patient fits the right criteria. I am interested in just what that criteria is. It seems like it is a moving criteria.

Dr. CHESON. What we try to find is patients for whom the cost-benefit ratio is in favor of the patient.

If you look at women with breast cancer, for example, the currently accepted situation is early in the disease, not a woman with metastatic disease. Early in the disease is a woman who at the time of her primary surgery is found to have 10 or more lymph nodes involved with tumor. Those women are found at such a high risk of recurring that it is felt the risks of this therapy are consistent with treating them in this approach.

As you develop more—as you see more favorable groups of patients whose likelihood of surviving with conventional therapy is quite high, then it may not be inappropriate treatment for those sorts of patients. One, for example, whose tumor is very small, has no lymph nodes involved and whose tumor exhibits a number of favorable characteristics, that would be considered favorable treatment.

As we learn more about the biology of the disease and as we are able to discover through clinical trials which patients are likely to benefit and which patients are not likely to benefit, that is where it helps us distinguish amongst those patients to offer the therapy to or those patients for whom something else might be more appropriate.

Mr. MYERS. Does the stage of the tumor or the dependence on hormone have any influence on the decision?

Dr. CHESON. Both the stage and the hormone dependency enter into the decision as to whether to offer this treatment.

In general, women with metastatic disease who have had a long period before they recurred, whose tumor is positive for what we call estrogen receptors, many physicians would offer those women hormonal therapy before the autologous bone marrow transplant. This may change as we learn more and more about different subsets of patients. It does depend on the stage, the extent of the disease, as well as the hormone status.

Mr. MYERS. At which end of the stage—Stage I versus Stage IV—would you treat?

Dr. CHESON. Well, I think more women are being treated with Stage IV disease and few women with Stage I. The second most common probably would be Stage II because of its lower incidence than Stage III, Stage IV being metastatic disease, Stage II having involved axillary lymph nodes.

Mr. MYERS. One witness testified this morning 10 or more tumors, 10 or more nodes that—do you use the standard of 10?

Dr. CHESON. Our clinical trials are based on 10. Now, there are other studies which are ongoing which are looking at the efficacy of this therapy in patients with seven to 10 nodes, seven to nine nodes, in women who have other unfavorable features, based on the biology of their particular tumor, certain characteristics.

Mr. MYERS. Does age have some factor in the determination? Being a senior citizen, I am asking that question.

Dr. CHESON. We are not allowed by the FDA to use chronological age as a discriminative of who is allowed in clinical trials.

Mr. MYERS. Is there another factor besides chronological age?

Dr. CHESON. Well, there is physiological age, the organ function, the general health of a particular patient which helps you decide whether they might tolerate the procedure or not.

Mr. MYERS. What research is being done today on storage of one's own bone marrow once cancer has been determined?

Dr. CHESON. That is what we are talking about here, is autologous bone marrow transplantation.

Mr. MYERS. That is using it right away.

Dr. CHESON. This can be stored.

Mr. MYERS. You can——

Dr. CHESON. In fact, it generally is frozen immediately and used several months later.

Mr. MYERS. How about five years later?

Dr. CHESON. Well, it would depend on the disease setting.

In general, we don't need to do this because the use of peripheral blood stem cells is becoming more and more widely utilized, and those are there when you need them. In addition, there are some clinical situations in which patients are really not likely to recur, and, therefore, it is not a good use of resources to store everybody's bone marrow if a chance of cure is extremely high.

Mr. MYERS. Well, if a person has been diagnosed with cancer, once they have—it has been put in remission and at that point you would not advise a patient to go ahead and stone their own bone marrow?

Dr. CHESON. It would depend on the setting. If it was a patient with acute leukemia who had a certain chromosome abnormality that portended an ominous outcome, that is a patient you could probably justify storing their bone marrow. However, for most patients with solid tumors, the use of peripheral blood stem cells, as I said, is becoming more widely used.

We are now developing new techniques of separating out these stem cells, which are evolving extremely rapidly, so that subjecting the patient to less in the way of harvesting procedures, you can get more stem cells to repopulate them. So when they finally need this, there are probably other less expensive, less noxious and more successful ways of getting the stem cell.

It is not the bone marrow we are looking for. It is the stem cells within the bone marrow. And those are also present in sufficient numbers in the blood.

Mr. MYERS. Then after a patient has found recurrence and you can take the bone marrow and extract the stems from it at that point then during that point?

Dr. CHESON. That can be done at that point. Either from the bone marrow, if it is not involved with cancer, or from the peripheral blood.

Mr. MYERS. What about bone cancer? Would that still be able to——

Dr. CHESON. It depends on which sort of bone cancer we are talking about. This therapy is being widely used for a form of bone marrow cancer called multiple myeloma, as well as forms of leukemia.

As far as tumors of bone, what we generally find is that tumors that are not responsive to standard chemotherapy, such as bone cancers, sarcomas, and so forth, tend not to benefit from this form of therapy. There has to be some responsiveness to standard doses of therapy in a particular type of tumor in general before it is regarded as being a candidate for high-dose therapy.

Mr. MYERS. Are you conducting any research on storage of umbilical cord fluid?

Dr. CHESON. There was just a hearing on that yesterday, as a matter of fact.

Mr. MYERS. Here someplace?

Dr. CHESON. Yeah.

Mr. MYERS. Missed that one.

Dr. CHESON. One of the congressmen from Brooklyn conducted a hearing yesterday on that very issue. The use of cord blood is an interesting option which is just being explored. There have been very few cases who have received a transplant of cord blood.

First of all, you have to realize that the number of stem cells you can get from cord blood is—at our current state of technology is sufficient only to repopulate a smaller person, a child. So it is probably not applicable today for the use of adults.

Whether storing cord blood will be a viable option in the future is the subject of considerable study. We have a number of grants and contracts throughout the NIH, not just the National Cancer Institute, which are investigating just this possibility.

Mr. MYERS. If you were having a baby today, would you have your child's fluid stored or what? I am going to be a grandfather at the end of this month. Should I—is somebody doing the work now? Should we do that?

Dr. CHESON. No.

Mr. MYERS. You wouldn't.

Dr. CHESON. There are some companies that are actually offering this for a fee. People will do anything for a fee.

Would I do this? No, because the likelihood of developing a disease for which this would be the effective form of therapy is small. The likelihood that if you get that disease there won't be other therapies which are probably better reduces the number. So the chance of this being something the child would ever need is so low that you really couldn't store on every child being born and expect that it would be of value to even a minuscule fraction of those on whom you store it.

Mr. MYERS. If one out of nine women is going to experience breast cancer, considering all the other cancers, ovarian cancers, lung cancer, all of these diseases, is there some reason why we might want to do this if it is going to be successful?

Dr. CHESON. You can always store the bone marrow or you can always harvest the bone marrow once the disease has been diagnosed or the peripheral blood stem cells. It is not something you need to have stored and sitting around.

Like if, hopefully, I am healthy, I don't think I am going to go down and have my bone marrow stored just in case I might develop a disease for which it was a reasonable and appropriate therapy. I would wait until I developed that and evaluate my options and say, okay, this is appropriate. I will go to a cancer center which is doing good research on the subject and then they can either take my bone marrow, my peripheral blood, they can use enriched stem cells from my peripheral blood or whatever sort of technology is au courant at that particular time.

Mr. MYERS. OPM, Mr. Smith, on page four you say, our position with respect to coverage for ABMT is based on its general acceptance in the medical community for each particular diagnosis. Some of the testimony today didn't come out that way. Can you explain why these other patients didn't have that experience? Their oncologists said this is the—they need it, the only thing that is going to keep them alive. Is there anything more determinate than that or more definitive?

Mr. SMITH. Yes, sir. And we have looked particularly to NCI to tell us when this particular therapy crosses over and becomes standard accepted medical practice, and it has not done that. As we have heard today, it is showing some promise, but it is not yet in that category of things that are standard medical practice that we automatically cover.

Mr. MYERS. Okay. I was reading somewhat different. You were going to give us information how long testicular cancer has been included.

My understanding, the Indiana School of Medicine, they tell me out there testicular cancer is curable without any recurrence if it is caught in the early enough stages. Is that one of the reasons why then you are approving testicular—is there some suggestion, the gender factor, the reason we were taking care of men and forgetting our daughters?

Mr. SMITH. Well, yes. And let me speak to two pieces of your question.

We have not told carriers they cannot cover things. The question for us is what things should we make them cover, rather than leaving it to their discretion. And we don't make them cover things that are——

Mr. MYERS. No carrier is going to cover anything that they don't have to, are they?

Mr. SMITH. Well, they do, yes. They do. Some of them drag their feet. Some of them are quicker about it. And I don't know what drives those things. Sometimes you have to hurry them along, and that is what we watch for.

On the gender issue, we cover ovarian, for example, German cell cancers, treatments with ABMT, as well as testicular. So it is important to me that the subcommittee understand that there aren't decisions here based on sex or gender. These are decisions based on scientific and medical sorts of issues.

Mr. MYERS. How about taxol treatment for ovarian cancer? Does OPM approve this?

Mr. SMITH. I believe taxol is accepted standard treatment now. Can you help me, Dr. Cheson?

Dr. CHESON. Yes. It is approved by the FDA for the treatment of ovarian and breast cancer. So, hopefully, there wouldn't be a problem with that.

Mr. SMITH. On the drug side, too, let me just say as a general program matter we cover everything that FDA approves because you have that very neat——

Mr. MYERS. It is their fault. You can sit aside and blame them for not approving.

How about synthesized taxol? Do you approve synthesized that they are developing now as well as taxol? Does it make any difference which taxol agent is used?

Dr. CHESON. Probably not.

Mr. MYERS. I have no other questions I will put in the record. Thank you very much, Madam Chairman.

Ms. NORTON. Thank you, Mr. Myers.

Mr. Smith and Dr. Cheson, were either of you aware that the Veterans Administration and medicaid pay for this treatment?

Mr. SMITH. I don't know about the Veterans Administration. Medicaid, I believe, is a State-by-State decision. I am also aware that Medicare does not, for example——

Mr. MYERS. Medicare does not?

Mr. SMITH. Medicare does not pay for ABMT for breast cancer.

Ms. NORTON. Dr. Cheson?

Dr. CHESON. That was my impression, but I am not as familiar with those sorts of things.

Ms. NORTON. Mr. Smith, indeed both of you, you see the difficulty here for the Congress when some of its programs, indeed directly out of taxpayers' funds, pay for this treatment and some of its agents do not? Do you recommend that that kind of distinction continue? Or would you like to see a single policy, Federal policy?

Mr. SMITH. I can certainly see some attraction to a single policy, but let me try to put it in a little bit different context.

I think the really important question facing the subcommittee and perhaps the whole Congress on the issue of health reform is are we going to cover, through health insurance, all experiments and investigations around medical treatments? Right now, we were in a position where we said none. I mean, the other extreme, of course, is that insurance will cover them all.

Ms. NORTON. Yes.

Mr. SMITH. If you are not in all——

Ms. NORTON. I am not going to allow you to pose a question in that simple-minded fashion. We are dealing with medical science that has now shown that it can move rapidly and that there are many shades in between the simple-minded polarization straw man notion you have just presented us. If that is what all that was, we wouldn't need this hearing in the first place.

What we are trying to do in the most analytic fashion is to face one of those gray areas and to ask how gray it has to be before we move toward what could be a lifesaving treatment. So I wish you would speak in those terms. Because we have already eliminated the polar extremes that you have just described.

Mr. SMITH. I am sorry, and I wanted to take this right where you were headed. I mean, I set the polar up there as kind of the easy thing to look at, and we are not there anymore.

You are precisely right. And the question for the subcommittee and I think for the country in health insurance is where are we going to draw that line now. And I don't have an easy answer to that. But we have relied on the scientific community to help us decide when things have crossed over and ought to be required by us from all of our plans.

Ms. NORTON. Your reliance on the scientific community—I want to ask Dr. Cheson about this as well. The language in your testimony is bone chilling to a woman. "No consensus", Mr. Smith says in his testimony, in the medical community. And yet we heard— we have heard evidence of what Sloan, the top-rated institution does. No consensus, and yet insurance carriers that don't shell out money easily these days, are, in fact, paying for this treatment outside of the Federal sector. Virginia says you got to pay for it. "No consensus" is what your testimony says.

Dr. Cheson uses a word in his testimony that also makes one wonder about what it would take: "more data is needed to definitively establish." Well, before it is definitively established, is there not some point where one would say, given other treatments and their ineffectiveness and the increasing effectiveness of that, we may not be definitive yet, but it is worth allowing a greater number of women to have access to this treatment? I am worried about the language both of you use, because it assures us that you are using a standard that is years off and Dr. Cheson doesn't even tell us how many years off. He says it will be several more years.

I want to tell you, in addition, that is a very unscientific term, "several". How many years? And what in the world do you mean by "consensus"? In this Congress, when we say consensus, we mean everybody agrees, unanimous consent. And definitively, my God, by that we mean that there can be no doubt.

Is that what both of you are talking about before women get access to this treatment? Shall we—shall we believe what the language in your testimony says, that this may happen not in the lifetime of many women who are out there now because there won't be a "consensus" of that definitive type?

Let me hear your answer. Yes?

Dr. CHESON. This procedure is available at many institutions around the country.

Ms. NORTON. Despite the absence of consensus?

Dr. CHESON. Despite the absence of consensus. We support its use in the clinical trial setting, not necessarily the randomized trials that are taking several years more. And I can't say how long because their rate of accrual is actually increasing as more and more institutions are participating.

Ms. NORTON. And yet Georgetown cannot get reimbursed from OPM for this because—outside of its clinical trials, even though it has its NCI treatment center. You, Mr. Smith, through the OPM, are not willing to say go ahead, even though it is the kind of setting that NCI approves.

Mr. SMITH. We have not to date gone beyond the national studies.

Ms. NORTON. Why? That is a perfectly approved setting. Why? Sloan, Georgetown, why won't you pay for somebody who goes to Sloan?

Mr. SMITH. Well—and we need to consider that. My answer, I think, was careful that we have not to date gone beyond the national NCI trials as we have moved for the first time into financing this sort of treatment.

Ms. NORTON. Mr. Smith, can I get your agreement that OPM will now look at going beyond NCI trials to consider the use of settings approved by NCI but not involved—not necessarily involved in randomized trials?

Mr. SMITH. I think that, yes, I think we need to commit to you to looking at that.

Ms. NORTON. Thank you.

Would both of you indicate, going back to my prior question, what you mean by the use of language that is as absolute as your testimony indicates? "Consensus", there is a plain meaning of language like that to those of us who understand English. "Definitively", those things say to us that promising treatments would be out of the question because they are not yet definitive. I wish you would explain yourselves.

Dr. CHESON. Definitively would refer to the results in these randomized study which statistical studies will tell us one treatment is better or not better than the other treatment.

Ms. NORTON. And, at the moment, you cannot say that this treatment is better than other treatments now in use?

Dr. CHESON. Right.

Ms. NORTON. Is it as good as other treatments now in use?

Dr. CHESON. It is likely as good as other treatments now in use.

The caveat I am throwing in there is because it is more toxic than other treatments in use. While its efficacy may be comparable, its toxicity may be greater, and there is the trade-off there that we are—which you look at in clinical trials.

Ms. NORTON. And when you say toxic——

Dr. CHESON. Toxicity.

Ms. NORTON. Toxicity, you don't necessarily mean death?

Dr. CHESON. I am referring to death, also.

Ms. NORTON. That is included in toxicity?

Dr. CHESON. Toxicity.

Ms. NORTON. In your testimony you say 40 to 50 percent die. It is interesting you give me figures in the past. How about the present?

Dr. CHESON. It depends if you go to an institution with a lot of experience, such as Sloan.

Ms. NORTON. What are those figures?

Dr. CHESON. Those figures are probably in the range of 5 percent or less.

Ms. NORTON. I wish you would have included those figures in your testimony.

Dr. CHESON. Dr. Champlin has planned on giving you those figures. But when it is performed by institutions who lack this expertise, that are not experienced in conducting this, it is still in the range of 20 to 30 percent.

Ms. NORTON. If you wanted to make this treatment available, Dr. Cheson, could you control for those factors, Podunk physicians and the rest? You could say—you could recommend to the Georgetowns and the Sloans of this world, to the OPM's of this world, that you yourself should—you yourself should not require this treatment unless the physician has a certain kind of experience.

Dr. CHESON. We don't have that capability.

Ms. NORTON. Well, they are depending on you. You just told me it is okay for Sloan and Georgetown, but it is not okay for less experienced people. Now you opt out of even your own recommendation. I want to know if these folks say, hey, NCI tells us what to do, then you say NCI doesn't know.

Dr. CHESON. That would be great, but we don't have the power to do that. That is not within our mandate to control the utility of this procedure.

Ms. NORTON. What is your mandate? What do you recommend to OPM? They told me that they depend on you. They told us.

Dr. CHESON. What we recommend to them is what we recommend to other care providers, is that therapies such as this should be reimbursed in the context of peer review clinical trials, not necessarily Phase III trials, which are randomized trials, but even earlier, since we feel that everybody has a role in improving the therapies to cancer patients.

Ms. NORTON. You wouldn't have any problem if OPM decided to allow these treatments in NCI-treatment-approved treatment institutions?

Dr. CHESON. We would welcome it.

Ms. NORTON. So with both of you at the table, Mr. Smith, you understand that NCI, whom you pass off to, has not vetoed your requiring this to be paid—this treatment to be paid by institutions that perform NCI treatment.

Mr. SMITH. And I had agreed earlier that we owe you a look at whether or not we should expand the definition of clinical trial in which we pay. And NCI's recommendation will be important. We look to them, I should say, as a caution, for the medical and scientific basis for what we should do but welcome their advice on the reimbursement as well.

Ms. NORTON. If this hearing has accomplished nothing else, your willingness to consider institutions that are NCI-treatment-recommended facilities takes us a step ahead, and we recognize that you are merely considering it.

Moreover, I just want to make it clear that as much as we press you—and that is our job—it is through examination and cross-examination, rather than to direct what should be done when scientific procedures and evidence recommends the opposite. This committee does not now and will never attempt to tell Dr. Cheson what to do. He has to be left to procedures that have a higher authority than this committee or the entire Congress.

But, Mr. Smith, we are confronted with what can be called for Federal employees disparate treatment when we see insurance carriers are willing to approve this treatment outside the Federal plan and not inside the Federal plan. When you have that kind of disparate treatment, it may not be discrimination, it may be perfectly reasonable, but the burden is on OPM to establish the reasonableness of the exclusion.

I will ask you, when do you think you can report in writing to this committee—subcommittee—on the outcome of your consideration of the use of requiring treatment in facilities that are NCI-treatment-approved facilities?

Mr. SMITH. That is a hard question for me to answer just on the spot because we haven't even begun the exploration of that, and we need to look at a number of things. Does a couple of months sound unreasonable?

Ms. NORTON. A couple months is reasonable.

Mr. SMITH. I think we should be able to do that.

Ms. NORTON. In other words, we would expect to receive the OPM reply by no later than the day that the recess is over. It would be early September. That will give—wait a minute.

Mr. SMITH. You cut me back to a month.

Ms. NORTON. I am sorry. Before our adjournment. Yeah, how about—how about two months from today? I am not trying to be cute with the dates.

[The information referred to follows:]

CONGRESS OF THE UNITED STATES,
HOUSE OF REPRESENTATIVES,
Washington, DC, August 12, 1994.

Hon. JAMES KING,
Director, Office of Personnel Management, Washington, DC.

DEAR MR. KING: We want to follow-up on a commitment made by Curtis Smith, OPM Associate Director for Retirement and Insurance, to review OPM's policy of restricting insurance coverage of bone marrow transplant treatment for breast cancer. Mr. Smith indicated to us that OPM would decide within two months whether to expand coverage to include all clinical trials of ABMT therapy.

During yesterday's hearing before the Subcommittee on Compensation and Employee Benefits, Dr. Bruce Cheson, Head of the National Cancer Institute's (NCI) Division of Cancer Treatment, testified that the NCI does not support OPM's decision to limit insurance coverage for autologous bone marrow transplantation (ABMT) for breast cancer to patients in "randomized" clinical trails only.

Dr. Cheson's testimony contradicts earlier testimony by Curtis Smith, who said, "We maintain close contact with the National Cancer Institute and they emphatically advise that ABMT therapy for breast cancer should not be performed outside of the clinical trial setting."

The key point brought out in the hearing is that there are different kinds of clinical trials approved by the National Cancer Institute. OPM reimburses only the randomized—or coinflip—trials, while NCI advocates reimbursement for *all* NCI approved trials, including non-coinflip trials.

The NCI approved non-coinflip trials, conducted at centers like Duke University and the University of Colorado, have shown extremely promising results. According to Dr. Roy Jones, Director of the Bone Marrow Transplant Program at the University of Colorado, the five-year relapse-free survival for high-risk primary breast cancer treated with ABMT is 35 percent better than any result reported in the medical literature by any research group using any conventional treatment.

The Virginia legislature, for example, recently passed a bill requiring every health insurance company to offer ABMT coverage for breast cancer.

Federal employees in Virginia, however, will not be covered. In Colorado, Blue Cross/Blue Shield will pay for the treatment for most private sector employees, but federal employees in Colorado are denied such coverage.

We are also deeply concerned about testimony received at the hearing from Attorney Arlene Grouch. She testified that OPM has colluded with FEHBP insurance carriers to undermine the enrollees' ability to obtain judicial review of carrier decisions rejecting claims for reimbursement. She indicated that OPM has negotiated an addendum to carrier contracts which provides that enrollees must appeal coverage determinations to OPM. She claims that OPM routinely sides with the carrier, and that when an enrollee subsequently brings suit against the carrier, the court, pursuant to the Administrative Procedures Act, must give deference to the agency's determination. The enrollee's case is then dismissed. While Ms. Grouch's claim has yet to be substantiated, we nonetheless believe it warrants investigation.

The contractual requirement appears to place a significant limitation on enrollee rights. We ask that you immediately provide us with information on the number, nature, and outcome of all enrollee appeals during FY 1993 and FY 1994. In addition, please provide a copy of the contract language addressing claims appeals.

Sincerely,

PATRICIA SCHROEDER,
ELEANOR HOLMES NORTON.

U.S. HOUSE OF REPRESENTATIVES,
COMMITTEE ON POST OFFICE AND CIVIL SERVICE,
Washington, DC, August 16, 1994.

Hon. JAMES B. KING,
Director, Office of Personnel Management, Washington, DC.

DEAR DIRECTOR KING: I am writing to confirm that OPM is, in fact, considering expanding its current insurance coverage to include patients in *all* National Cancer Institute (NCI) approved clinical trials of a promising new breast cancer treatment—high-dose chemotherapy with autologous bone marrow transplantation (HDC/ABMT). In an important development from the hearing last Thursday of my Subcommittee on Compensation and Employee Benefits, OPM Associate Director Curtis Smith committed that OPM would reconsider *within two months*—that is, by *October 11, 1994*—its policy of limiting coverage to patients in an extremely small number of "randomized" clinical trials only. Particularly in light of NCI testimony that there was no reason that patients should not be treated through NCI-approved treatment facilities, such as Georgetown University Hospital and Sloan Kettering, the Subcommittee would anticipate that OPM would require coverage of appropriate breast cancer patients.

Your agency's action in allowing greater access to cancer treatment by often desperate women would be a highly significant and humane development. However, in light of the testimony of federal employees whose lives have apparently been saved by this therapy but whose applications for reimbursement were denied by their insurance carriers, it would have been remarkable and cruel if OPM had adhered to its original position of refusing to consider expanding access to this life-saving treatment until randomized trials were completed. There is significant evidence that already in some trials, HDC/ABMT has proved considerably more effective than conventional treatment. Considering the seriousness of past denials, the life and death implications of your review, and the position of NCI (on which Mr. Smith says you rely) that access should be expanded, I urge you to revise your current policy without delay *even before the October 11 deadline.*

When an experimental treatment is shown in trials to have higher success rates than conventional chemotherapy, it would seem the height of callousness to impose bureaucratic obstacles that effectively deny women the chance to participate in approved programs that might well save their lives. I hope that, in revisiting the question of coverage of HDC/ABMT by FEHBP insurance carriers, you will recognize the impact your decisions have had and will continue to have on the health and well-being of women employees and their families.

May I ask also that you respond to testimony and reports of possible collusion between OPM and FEHBP insurance carriers aimed at undermining enrollees' ability to obtain judicial review of their rejected claims for reimbursement of HDC/ABMT treatment. Successful court challenges of HDC/ABMT coverage decisions by federal employees appear to have precipitated specific new carrier provisions, approved by OPM, that arbitrarily bar coverage for HDC/ABMT. After employees achieved the right to coverage in court, a new contractual addendum appeared in FEHBP insurance policies that requires FEHBP enrollees to appeal all coverage determinations directly to OPM. This new requirement has given the appearance of collusion because OPM routinely sides with the insurance carrier and because courts are legally required to defer to OPM's determination.

I ask you to provide my Subcommittee with information on the number, nature, and outcome of all enrollee appeals of FEHBP claims during FY 1993 and FY 1994 within 30 days of the hearing—that is, by September 12, 1994. In addition, please provide a copy of the contract language addressing claims appeals.

Sincerely,

ELEANOR HOLMES NORTON.

U.S. OFFICE OF PERSONNEL MANAGEMENT,
OFFICE OF THE DIRECTOR,
Washington, DC, September 28, 1994.

Hon. ELEANOR HOLMES NORTON,
U.S. House of Representatives, Washington, DC.

DEAR DELEGATE NORTON: Thank you for your letters of August 12, 1993, and August 16, 1994, concerning issues discussed during the Subcommittee on Compensation and Employee Benefits' hearing on High Dose Chemotherapy/Autologous Bone Marrow Transplants. We are pleased to advise you of the status of OPM's commitment to consider expanding coverage to include HDC/ABMT for breast cancer and to comply with your requests for additional information.

We have decided to require all FEHB plans to provide coverage immediately for HDC/ABMT for the treatment of breast cancer, multiple myeloma and epithelial ovarian cancer in addition to diagnoses for which it is considered standard treatment. At a minimum, the plans must provide coverage for non-randomized clinical trials. This requirement will apply to all FEHB plans, both fee-for-service and HMO's.

You indicated a deep concern about the testimony presented by Attorney Arlene Grouch with regard to OPM's disputed claims process. Rather than undermining the enrollees' ability to obtain judicial review, the disputed claims process provides an alternative vehicle whereby the enrollee can appeal a carrier denial. The process does not preclude an enrollee from going to court. It simply provides an effective interim step. If OPM should determine that the benefit or service is due, it requires the carrier to provide the payment or the service. In the aggregate, more than one third of the enrollees who come to OPM for disputed claims review have the carriers' decisions overturned as is shown in the following table.

Year	Claims processed	Carrier decisions overturned
1993	8174	2650
1994—through July	3361	1170

Claims are not categorized by diagnosis or treatment but rather by the nature of the dispute as described by the enrollee. The majority of the disputed claims fall into the following categories: Fee Dispute; Non-covered Hospital Confinement; Not Medically Necessary; Care Not in Accordance with Accepted Medical Standards; Dental; Non-covered Provider; Medical Emergency; Physical, Speech, and Occupational Therapy; Prescription Drugs; and Precertification/Preauthorization.

The disputed claims regulation was revised in 1986 to improve the administration of the disputed claims process by specifying the steps in the process and adding timeframes for each step. The disputed claims language for both the contracts and the brochures was amended most recently for the 1993 contract year. I have enclosed copies of both the standard contract language (Section 2.3 (h) and (i)) and the brochure language (1994 Blue Cross/Blue Shield brochure) as an addendum. Since courts almost always remand the case to OPM if we have not issued a decision, the language has been modified to more specifically describe the process so that enrollees will not lose time if they decide to pursue litigation. The revision of the regulation and the modifications of contract and brochure language reflect improvements in the administrative process and OPM's intent to provide specific information in the interest of improved customer service.

The enclosed addendum includes the information you requested. However, if you should require any additional information, please do not hesitate to contact me.

Sincerely,

JAMES B. KING,
Director,

Enclosure.

SECTION 2.3   PAYMENT OF BENEFITS AND PROVISION OF SERVICE AND SUPPLIES
(JANUARY 1991)

(a) By enrolling or accepting services under this contract, Members are obligated to all terms, conditions, and provisions of this contract. The Carrier may request Members to complete reasonable forms or provide information which the Carrier may reasonably request; provided, however, that the Carrier shall not require Members to complete any form as a precondition of receiving benefits unless the form has first been approved for use by OPM. Forms requiring specific approval do not include claim forms and other forms necessary to receive payment of individual claims.

(b) All benefits shall be paid by draft within a reasonable time after receipt of reasonable proof covering the occurrence, character, and extent of the event for which the claim is made. The claimant shall furnish satisfactory evidence that all services or supplies for which expenses are claimed are covered services or supplies within the meaning of the contract.

(c) The procedures and time period for filing claims shall be as specified in the brochure. However, failure to file a claim within the time required shall not in itself invalidate or reduce any claim where timely filing was prevented by administrative operations of Government or legal incapacitation, provided the claim was submitted as soon as reasonably possible.

(d) The Carrier may request a Member to submit to one or more medical examinations to determine whether benefits applied for are for services and supplies necessary for the diagnosis or treatment of an illness or injury of the Member and may withhold payment of such benefits pending completion of the examinations. The examinations will be made at the expense of the Carrier by a physician selected by the Member from a panel of at least three physicians whose names are furnished by the Carrier, and the results of the examinations will be made available to the Carrier and the Member.

(e) As a condition precedent to the provision of benefits hereunder, the Carrier, to the extent reasonable and necessary and consistent with Federal law, shall be entitled to obtain from any person, organization or Government agency, including the Office of Personnel Management, all information and records relating to visits or examination of, or treatment rendered or supplies furnished to, a Member as the Carrier requires in the administration of such benefits. The Carrier may obtain from any insurance company or other organization or person any information, with respect to any Member, which it has determined is reasonably necessary to:

(1) Identify enrollment in a plan,

(2) Verify eligibility for payment of a claim for health benefits, and

(3) Carry out the provisions of the contract, such as subrogation, recovery of payments made in error, workers compensation, and coordination of benefits.

(f) Benefits are payable to the Enrollee in the Plan or his or her assignees. However, under the following circumstances different payment arrangements are allowed:

(1) If benefits become payable to the estate of an Enrollee or an Enrollee is a minor, or an Enrollee is physically or mentally not competent to give a valid release, the Carrier may either pay such benefits directly to a hospital or other provider of services or pay such benefits to any relative by blood or connection by marriage of the Enrollee determined by the Carrier to be equitably entitled thereto.

(2) Reimbursement Payments. If dependent children, covered as family members under a self-and-family enrollment, are in the custody of a person other than the person maintaining the enrollment, and if that other person certifies to the Carrier that he or she has custody of and financial responsibility for the dependent children, then reimbursement by the Carrier for any covered medical service or supply shall be made to that person. This requirement may be varied by mutual agreement between the Enrollee and the person having custody of the dependent children, or by an order of a court of competent jurisdiction.

(3) Any payments made in good faith in accordance with paragraphs (f)(1) and (f)(2) will fully discharge the Carrier to the extent of such payment.

(g) If the Carrier or OPM determines that a Member's claim has been paid in error for any reason, the Carrier shall make a diligent effort to recover such overpayment from the Member or the provider. If the Carrier is unable to recover the erroneous payment, the Carrier may recover erroneous payments to the Member by reducing his or her future benefits or recover erroneous payment to the provider by reducing the provider's future reimbursements for claims incurred by the same Member.

(h) No lawsuit may be brought by or on behalf of a Member to recover on a claim for Plan benefits until the Member or, in the case of an assigned claim, the Member's provider exhausts this OPM review procedure which is established at section 890.105, Title 5, Code of Federal Regulations (CFR). If OPM upholds the Carrier decision on the Member's claim, and the Member then decides to bring a lawsuit based on the claim denial, the lawsuit must be brought no later than December 31 of the third year after the year in which the services or supplies upon which the claim is predicated were provided. Pursuant to section 890.107, Title 5, CFR, such a lawsuit must be brought against the Carrier.

(i) Federal law exclusively governs all Member claims for relief in a lawsuit that relate to Plan benefits or coverage provided to Members or payments with respect to those benefits. As provided under this agreement between the Carrier and the Office of Personnel Management, judicial action on such claims for relief is limited to a review of OPM's final decision to determine if it is arbitrary or capricious under the terms of the brochure statement of benefits. Damages recoverable in such lawsuits are limited to the amount of Plan contract benefits in dispute, plus simple prejudgment interest (at the rate prescribed by section 1961(a) of title 28, U.S. Code) and court costs.

Section 2.4 Termination of Coverage and Conversion Privileges (January 1991)

(a) A Member's coverage is terminated as specified in regulations issued by the OPM. Benefits after termination of coverage are as specified in the regulations.

(b) A Member is entitled to a temporary continuation of coverage or an extension of coverage under the conditions and to the extent specified in the regulations.

(c) A Member whose coverage hereunder has terminated is entitled, upon application within the times and under the conditions specified in regulations, to a nongroup contract regularly offered for the purpose of conversion from the contractor or similar contracts. The conversion contract shall be in compliance with 5 U.S.C., chapter 89, and regulations issued thereunder.

(d) Costs associated with writing or providing benefits under conversion contracts shall not be an allowable cost of this contract.

(e) The Carrier will maintain on file with OPM copies of the conversion policies offered to persons whose coverage under this contract terminates and advise OPM promptly of any changes in the policies. The Contracting Officer may waive this requirement where because of the large number of different conversion policies offered by the Carrier it would be impractical to maintain a complete up-to-date file of all policies. In this case the Carrier shall submit a representative sample of the general types of policies offered and provide copies of specific policies on demand.

Section 2.5 Subrogation (January 1991)

The Carrier's subrogation rights, procedures and policies, including recovery rights, shall be in accordance with the provisions of the brochure.

Section 2.6 Coordination of Benefits (January 1991) (FEHBAR)

(a) The Carrier shall coordinate the payment of benefits under this contract with the payment of benefits under Medicare, other group health benefits coverages, and the payment of medical and hospital costs under no-fault or other automobile insurance that pays benefits without regard to fault.

(b) The Carrier shall not pay benefits under this contract until it has determined whether it is the primary carrier or unless permitted to do so by the Contracting Officer.

(c) In coordinating benefits between plans, the Carrier shall follow the order of precedence established by the NAIC Model Guidelines for Coordination of Benefits (COB) as specified by OPM.

(d) Where (1) the Carrier makes payments under this contract which are subject to COB provisions; (2) the payments are erroneous, not in accordance with the terms of the contract, or in excess of the limitations applicable under this contract; and (3) the Carrier is unable to recover such COB overpayments from the Member or the providers of services or supples, the Contracting Officer may allow such amounts to be charged to the contract; the Carrier must be prepared to demonstrate that it has made a diligent effort to recover such COB overpayments.

How to Claim Benefits

DISPUTED CLAIMS

If a claim for payment or service is denied, the Plan will reconsider its denial on receipt of a written request within one year of the denial. The written request should state, in terms of applicable brochure provisions, the reasons you believe that the denied claim for payment or service should have been paid or provided. Within 30 days after receipt of your request for reconsideration, the Plan must affirm the denial in writing to you, pay the claim, provide the service, or request additional information reasonably necessary to make a determination. If this information is not supplied within 60 days, the Plan will base its decision on the information it has on hand.

If the Plan affirms its denial, you have a right to a review by OPM to determine whether the Plan has acted in accordance with its contract in adjudicating the claim. Keep these things in mind before seeking OPM review:

Submit bills from providers for payment to the Plan along with the appropriate claim form; do not send bills to the address below or any other office within OPM except in connection with a disputed claim.

Providers, legal counsel, and other interested parties may use this procedure only on behalf of an with the specific written consent of the member, and are required to demonstrate that the member has assigned all of his or her rights to the provider with regard to that particular claim.

First check with your provider of facility to be sure that the Plan was billed correctly; for instance, that the correct procedure code was used, complications were correctly indicated on the billing or operative report, etc. As shown on pages 7 and 8, Covered charges are determined and controlled solely by the Plan and are based upon information available to it.

If you request an OPM review, you must send a copy of the Plan's reconsideration decision.

OPM review may be obtained by writing to: Office of Personnel Management, Retirement and Insurance Group, Office of Insurance Programs, Disputed Claims Branch III, P.O. Box 436, Washington, DC 20044.

OPM must receive a request for review, along with a copy of your letter to the Plan and its reply, within 90 days of the Plan's affirmation of the denial.

You may ask OPM for a review if the Plan fails to respond within 30 days of your written request for reconsideration or 30 days after you have supplied additional information. In this case, OPM must receive a request for review within 120 days of your request to the Plan for reconsideration or the date you were notified that the Plan needed additional information. In you request for review, show (a) the date of your request to the Plan, or (b) the dates the Plan requested and you provided additional information to the Plan.

No lawsuit may be brought to recover on a claim for Service Benefit Plan benefits until you or, in the case of an assigned claim, your provider exhausts this OPM review procedure which is established at section 890.105, title 5, Code of Federal Regulations (CFR). If OPM upholds the Local Plan's decision on your claim, and you then decide to bring a lawsuit based on the claim denial, the lawsuit must be brought no later than December 31 of the third year after the year in which the services or supplies upon which the claim is predicated were provided. Pursuant to section 890.107, title 5, CFR, such a lawsuit must be brought against the Local Plan that denied your claim.

Federal law exclusively governs all claims for relief in a lawsuit that relate to this Plan's benefits or coverage or payments with respect to those benefits. As provided under the agreement between the Blue Cross and Blue Shield Association and the Office of Personnel Management, judicial action on such claims for relief is limited to a review of OPM's final decision to determine if it is arbitrary or capricious under the terms of this statement of benefits in dispute, plus simple prejudgement interest (at the rate prescribed by section 1961(a) of title 28, U.S. Code) and court costs.

Privacy Act statement—If you ask OPM to review a denial of a claim for payment or service, OPM is authorized by chapter 89 of title 5, U.S. Code, to use the information collected from you and the Plan to determine if the Plan has acted properly in denying you the payment or service, and the information so collected may be disclosed to you and/or the Plan in support of OPM's decision on the disputed claim.

Ms. NORTON. Let me say to both of you, I appreciate the way you have accepted our grilling. It is meant in the spirit of trying to get an explanation as to what, in fact, has been behind your thinking. We appreciate hearing that thinking. You have heard some disagreement from this committee. We have appreciated understanding, having you lay out your thinking. We very much appreciate the spirit in which you come forward.

Mrs. Morella has come back. She may have more questions.

Mrs. MORELLA. You have done a great job, Madam Chair. I am sure they have enjoyed thoroughly being here at this subcommittee hearing. We certainly have learned a great deal and do appreciate you coming.

I just wanted to verify something I think I heard a while ago with regard to what OPM will have the carriers pay for in terms of the clinical trials. They flip a coin. Ones they pay for, the others they don't. Is there a distinction? Are there some trials they pay for and some that they don't, that they have had the carriers pay for?

Mr. SMITH. The ones that we are participating in now are the large national trials which are randomized. I think that is the flip-coin trials.

Mrs. MORELLA. Randomized.

Mr. SMITH. We have taken just that first step and have agreed to consider the next step.

Mrs. MORELLA. So there are some. The answer is, yes, there are some you do pay for and some you don't.

Mr. SMITH. That is correct.

Mrs. MORELLA. Therein is another inequity which says you should pay for them all. Thank you.

Ms. NORTON. Just let me ask you one question before you leave. The cost of this treatment—are there treatments of comparable cost that OPM routinely pays for?

Mr. SMITH. Certainly. Transplants. Most transplants are in this range. This issue has not come up before, but I would like to categorically say cost is not an issue here.

Ms. NORTON. That is very important for the record.

I notice the cost is costly, but I myself have seen—$60,000 or $70,000 and that is I think an average cost that has been told to us.

I know, of course, of costs well beyond that for people with diseases far less serious than cancer. You almost figure if you go to a hospital emergency room you will end up with that these days.

I thank you very much. Thanks to both of you very much.

Could we call the next panel, please? Dr. Roy B. Jones, Director of the Bone Marrow Transplant Program, University of Colorado. I am sorry. Dr. Richard Champlin, President of the American Society for Blood and Bone Marrow Transplants from Houston; and Dr. I. Craig Henderson, Director of the Clinical Center Program, University of San Francisco, California.

STATEMENTS OF DR. ROY B. JONES, DIRECTOR OF THE BONE MARROW TRANSPLANT PROGRAM, UNIVERSITY OF COLORADO; DR. RICHARD CHAMPLIN, PRESIDENT OF THE AMERICAN SOCIETY FOR BLOOD AND BONE MARROW TRANSPLANTS, HOUSTON; AND DR. I. CRAIG HENDERSON, DIRECTOR OF THE CLINICAL CENTER PROGRAM, UNIVERSITY OF SAN FRANCISCO

Ms. NORTON. We apologize that you had to wait so long. Such are the ways of subcommittees of the Congress. You may proceed in any order you desire.

Dr. HENDERSON. Thank you for the opportunity to testify here.

My name is Craig Henderson. I am a medical oncologist who treats patients with breast cancer, and over the past 20 years I have conducted numerous studies evaluating new treatments for breast cancer. I have been a part of several treatments evaluating high-dose chemotherapy and bone marrow transplant, including the first team that used this treatment at the Dana–Farber Cancer Institute under the direction of Emil Frei in 1974, as well as a team that is now running a large, multi-institutional randomized trial sponsored by the National Cancer Institute.

I am a Professor of Medicine and Chief of Oncology at the University of San Francisco, California. I chair the Cancer and Leukemia Group B. I have served on the Oncologic Drugs Committee of the FDA, and I chaired this committee for three years.

I have served on the technology assessment panels or been a consultant to various insurance companies or HMOs, including the technology assessment of Blue Cross and Kaiser of Southern California. In each of these instances, I have declined compensation to avoid any potential conflict of interest regarding these issues.

For many years now, we in the United States have had a very orderly process of evaluating potentially useful new drugs and devices. This involves a number of steps.

However, during all of the phases of tests in humans, we look for an effect of the treatment on the disease, but phase II studies are more specifically designed for this purpose. In most phase II studies, we treat the patients we think are most likely to benefit using the doses of drugs we have already determined to be optimal or the maximally tolerated in phase I studies.

In the case of anti-cancer drugs, we look for evidence that a lump we can feel on examination or see on an X-ray has shrunk in size. If there is no evidence that treatment has affected the tumor in these phase II studies, further research on the drug is usually abandoned.

At the end of phase II, we are able to state whether the treatment has any potential benefit in humans, but we cannot state that it is as effective or safe as other treatments of that disease. For this reason, we go on to the last phase of evaluation, phase III, in which the new treatment is compared to a standard therapy.

In some cases, phase III evaluation is done by comparing the results of a new treatment with results previously achieved using conventional therapy. However, this approach has often misled us in the past, and now we more often employ a randomized clinical trial in which half the patients receive the new treatment while the other half receive standard therapy.

Phase III trials involve many more patients, usually hundreds or thousands, and are more difficult and expensive to do. While it might seem simple to treat a patient with a new therapy and determine whether he/she feels better, the fact that the patient feels better may not be related to the treatment. This is because even ineffective treatments will often make a patient feel better. This is called the placebo effect. The placebo effect occurs even when the new treatment has quite a few side effects. However, before we routinely use a drug to treat cancer patients, we want to know that it has more than a placebo effect. Just because a drug causes a tumor to shrink, it does not always follow that the drug will relieve pain or other symptoms of cancer.

The same is true for prolonging life. Sometimes it is easy to determine if a drug will cure patients or at least make them live longer. Dr. Cheson gave an example. If you have a group of patients with an untreatable cancer that is invariably fatal in a short time, for example, six months, and a new treatment prolongs life so that all or almost all patients live longer, two years, it is easy to conclude is there is a benefit. Fortunately for patients and unfortunately for researchers and for science, it is not usually that simple, especially for diseases such as breast cancer. No treatment has yet been identified that will cure a breast cancer patient once the disease has spread to distant sites, such as lung, bone, liver or brain.

However, this does not mean the patient will die right away or even soon. Some patients will live for only a few months after the detection of distant spread. At least half will live for two to three years; and some will live for a decade or more after the disease has spread. A very few have been reported to live with distant metastases for 20 or 30 or even 40 years. Thus, if a doctor treats a small number of patients—20 or 30—and a few live for five years, how does he or she know they wouldn't have lived that long without the treatment or with more conventional therapy?

Before a new drug is approved by the FDA, it must go through all three phases of evaluation. Before any patient is enrolled, the trials must be approved by both the FDA and a local Human Protection Committee or institutional review board. Among the things that the Human Protection Committee evaluates most carefully is the informed consent document to ensure that patients who enroll in the study or any trial of an institution will be told all that is known about the benefits of this drug as well as the potential dangers.

Until the drug is approved by the FDA for general use, however, only those patients who are enrolled in these phase one, phase two, or phrase three trials can get the drug. Thus, we have a long-standing tradition in the United States of restricting the right of a physician to prescribe a drug or for a patient to have access to a drug until these studies are completed. We have been proud of the fact that this process has saved the American public from tragedies that occurred in countries with less stringent requirements for drug approval. The most striking example of such a tragedy was thalidomide, a drug used to alleviate the morning sickness associated with pregnancy. Many of the children born to women who took this drug were severely deformed.

Once a drug is approved by the FDA, however, we do not generally restrict the physician's right to prescribe a drug even at doses for conditions that were not originally described in the FDA approval. In addition, restrictions on the use of surgery and other procedures that do not come under the purview of the FDA have in the past been left to the discretion of the hospitals where these procedures were performed.

However, in the last 40 years, the number of new therapies and technologies developed by the medical profession and the pharmaceutical industry exceed by many fold the number introduced in any prior century of medical history. This has contributed to a rapid escalation in the cost of medical care. In some cases, it has also resulted in adding to, rather than alleviating, the suffering of our patients. This happens when a toxic therapy is accepted without adequate evaluation and is subsequently found to have no greater value than standard treatments.

It is increasingly happening as we order more and more tests which oftentimes are very uncomfortable for our patients.

High dose chemotherapy with autologous bone marrow transplant falls under the category of a treatment not requiring FDA approval. All of the drugs used in these high dose regimens have previously been approved for use at lower doses to treat either breast cancer or to treat other types of cancers. Since some of these drugs are known to be effective at low doses, thus it would have been very surprising if the phase two studies of high dose chemotherapy and bone marrow transplant had resulted in no tumor shrinkage in any of these patients. The important question—which has not been answered—is are the high doses of chemotherapy and bone marrow transplant as good as or better than conventional chemotherapy?

Most experts in the field of breast cancer and bone marrow transplant agree there is very little or no benefit from the use of this technique in patients whose breast cancer has grown while they are receiving conventional dose chemotherapy. In this morning's discussion, several people brought up the discussion of testicular cancer. This is a single indication and it is not generally approved for other indications. The most promising results are from studies in which patients have not been given prior chemotherapy to shrink these metastases. These are the tumor growths occurring throughout the body when breast cancer spreads from its original site in the breast. In most of the published studies, patients were given four to six months of conventional dose chemotherapy. If their tumor shrank as a result of conventional dose treatment, they were given one or two additional courses of high dose chemotherapy with bone marrow transplant. In these trials the percentage of patients whose tumors disappeared completely after this treatment was considerably higher than that reported in previous years using conventional dose chemotherapy. However—and this is a very important caveat to understanding the problems of the interpretation—the percentage of patients in these transplant studies whose tumor completely disappeared before the high dose chemotherapy was given was also much higher than previously reported from studies using the same conventional dose chemotherapy. This suggests that the patients enrolled in these transplant studies were in some way different than the patients enrolled in other trials. It is likely their disease was more responsive to chemotherapy.

Only six or seven of these trials published results of the survival of patients with metastatic breast cancer treated with high dose chemotherapy and bone marrow transplant. In these studies the average or median survival of a transplanted patient was no longer and might even be slightly shorter than that of patients treated with conventional chemotherapy. Similarly, the percentage of patients alive at two to five years following transplant was no greater than that achieved with the best conventional chemotherapy regimens. There is absolutely no evidence that any woman has been cured with high dose chemotherapy who would not have been cured with conventional therapy.

Several phase two studies have now been published—and they have been referred to this morning—as studies in patients with 10 or more positive nodes and several studies have been published for studies of treating patients whose cancer has not spread widely. These studies used high dose chemotherapy and bone marrow transplant as an adjuvant in patients with 10 or more positive nodes to suggest the chemotherapy may prolong the time until the cancer comes back in distant organs. None of these studies has shown this treatment will prolong the lives of these patients. As with the use of this treatment in patients with widespread disease, there is not yet evidence any of these patients have been cured with this therapy.

Tumors seem to disappear more completely following high dose chemotherapy and bone marrow transplant than following conventional therapy. At the same time, there is no evidence that treatment prolongs patient survival. In the face of this uncertainty about whether there really is a net benefit for using high dose chemotherapy and bone marrow transplant in any group of patients, we have initiated three nationwide randomized trials to evaluate this therapy. Almost all American leaders in the study of breast cancer have publicly endorsed these studies. Most of the prestigious institutions of this country have enrolled patients on these studies including Duke University, Johns Hopkins, Dana-Farber Cancer Institute at Harvard, the University of Pennsylvania, the University of Chicago, the University of Colorado, and the University of California at San Francisco. This is only a partial list. It would be unethical to run these trials if it were already known that high dose chemotherapy and bone marrow transplant were better than conventional chemotherapy.

Randomized trials frequently show a treatment thought to be promising in early trials is not as good as we had hoped. In the treatment of breast cancer, we have a very good example: the Halstead radical mastectomy. This form of surgery which removes the breast, all the muscles on the chest wall, skin overlying these muscles—thus requiring a skin graft— and many lymph nodes was our standard treatment for breast cancer during the first 70 years of this century. This form of surgery was more mutilating than the surgery used today or in the 19th Century. It was also more expensive, since it required the patient be in the operating room for a longer period of time; the surgeon had to be very skilled; and it took weeks for the patient to recover from the operation. Eventually, we were able to show in randomized trials this surgery was not associated with a longer life and did not cure more patients than less mutilating and less expensive surgical procedures. But this was only after five to seven million women had received this operation.

We had approximately 30 years of opposition to randomized trials before we finally were able to complete them. Like the radical mastectomy, high dose chemotherapy and bone marrow transplant makes sense to the average person. It is a powerful and technologically demanding approach to a problem that is difficult to understand and that strikes fear in the heart of every woman. It is a big solution to a big problem. For this reason, it is difficult for most patients to understand why they can only receive this treatment if they are in a trial. The orderly process of performing phase one, two, and three studies takes years. Most women with breast cancer do not feel they can wait that long. They frequently see this treatment as their only hope.

After years of practicing medicine, I am convinced that the single most important element contributing to a good quality of life is hope. Take away hope, and even the cured patient will suffer for the remainder of her life. But hope is not generated by facts and figures. It is the province of healers, whether it is a physician, a nurse, a priest or provider of a remedy outside the mainstream of medicine. Thus if anyone says to the patient your only hope for cure is high dose chemotherapy and bone marrow transplant, it is likely to haunt the patient until she has acted on this recommendation.

While making treatment decisions, breast cancer patients are extremely vulnerable. They want to make sure they have not overlooked a single opportunity and the media plays on this vulnerability. The results of relatively minor laboratory experiments are reported in our daily newspapers without a clear indication such experiments are not likely to affect the treatment of any human disease, and if they do lead to an effective treatment, it is not likely to be available for years or decades. Once instilled in a patient's heart, how can any of us—including judges or juries—take away that which the patient concluded correctly or incorrectly is her only hope.

In this charged atmosphere, it has been difficult for insurers to develop a policy regarding payment for high dose chemotherapy and bone marrow transplant. Those who pay for health insurance— most often businesses and government—demand that the escalating health care costs be controlled. One rational way to cut costs is to stop paying for therapies that are not effective.

Many insurance companies now require rigorous evidence that a treatment is truly safe and effective before paying for it, much as the FDA does before approving a new drug. When high dose chemotherapy and bone marrow transplant is assessed in this way, as the FDA would do, most insurers have found there are insufficient data to justify paying for this as standard treatment.

High dose chemotherapy and bone marrow transplant is a toxic and very costly treatment. Those who have concluded that it is the single best hope for a cure find it difficult not to feel that cost is the principal motivation of the insurer who denies coverage. Traditionally, insurance contracts have excluded payment for experimental therapies or investigational therapies, if you prefer.

However, if the insurer does not pay the medical costs of the patients who are in these trials, the trials will never be completed. Doctors who passionately believe in this treatment—that is in chemotherapy and bone marrow transplant—argue it is not experimental, hoping insurers will then allow them to prescribe the therapy or at least evaluate it further. In recent years, several insurers, including some of the—but not all—but some of the Blue Cross and Blue Shield plans, have sought to alleviate this problem by raising special funds to pay for the costs of their patients when enrolled in trials supported by the National Cancer Institute even if they don't pay the costs of this treatment outside of such trials.

How do we resolve this conflict between the humanistic desire to comfort the seriously ill and the scientific need to find out which treatments really work?

I am convinced it is not by abandoning rigorous assessment of new treatments. To do so will not only increase the cost of medicine, it will lead us down many blind alleys. In some cases—like that of the radical mastectomy—it may delay our search for better therapies for decades or even centuries. Instead, we need to pay for the treatment of any patient who participates in national clinical trials and speed up the process of evaluation so there is not such a long delay between the promise and the reality of a new therapy.

I will say parenthetically, however, that not all trials are equal. Recent experience of AIDS activists illustrate the importance of completing proper, usually randomized trials before making a therapy generally available. A decade ago, when AIDS activists first began to demand drugs be available to patients before trials were completed, accrual to some studies decreased substantially. This seemed to slow the process of finding a cure.

However, I recently participated in a meeting to assess data for a new drug to treat an AIDS-related tumor. Several AIDS activists participated in this meeting. I was impressed with how carefully and critically they examined the data. This was a contrast to what I had seen 10 years earlier. During the break I asked them how they arrived at this point. They answered "Watching thousands of our friends die in spite of our best efforts led us to realize there was more to this than just making the treatments available."

Thank you.

[The prepared statement of Dr. Henderson follows:]

PREPARED STATEMENT OF DR. I. CRAIG HENDERSON, DIRECTOR OF THE CLINICAL CENTER PROGRAM, UNIVERSITY OF SAN FRANCISCO

My name is Craig Henderson. I am a medical oncologist who treats patients with breast cancer, and over the past 20 years I have conducted numerous studies evaluating new treatments for breast cancer. I have been a part of several teams evaluating high dose chemotherapy and bone marrow transplant, including the first team that used this treatment at the Dana-Farber Cancer Institute under the direction of Dr. Emil Frei III in 1974 and a team now running a large, multi-institutional randomized trial. I am a Professor of Medicine and Chief of Medical Oncology at the University of California, San Francisco. I chair the Breast Cancer committee of the Cancer and Leukemia Group B. I have served on the Oncologic Drugs Committee of the FDA, and I chaired this committee for three years. I have served on the technology assessment panels or have been a consultant to various insurance companies or HMO's, including the technology assessment panel of the Blue Cross/Blue Shield National Association and Kaiser of Southern California. In each of these instances I have declined compensation to avoid any potential conflict of interest regarding these issues.

For many years now, we, in the United States, have had a very orderly process of evaluating potentially useful new drugs and devices. This involves a number of steps. The first of these are invariably performed in laboratories using cells in petri dishes or animals. From these experiments we can obtain some estimate of the proper doses of drugs that will be safe, the toxicities or side effects that the patient is likely to experience, and the likelihood that a drug will be effective against a particular disease. But these are only estimates.

The first tests in humans determine the doses of drugs that can be used safely. We always start with a dose quite a bit below those we think will ultimately prove to be most effective and then gradually increase the dose, observing the patients for both expected and unexpected toxicities. When we reach a dose just below that we believe will be intolerable or might be fatal, we back off and use a slightly lower dose in future studies. We refer to this series of studies as "phase I" in the development of a new treatment.

During all phases of testing we look for an effect of the treatment on the disease, but phase II studies are more specifically designed for this purpose. In most phase II studies we treat the patients we think are most likely to benefit, using the dose of drug determined to be optimal in phase I studies. In the case of anti-cancer drugs, we look for evidence that a lump we can feel on examination or see in an x-ray has shrunk in size. If there is no evidence that the treatment has affected the tumor in these phase II studies, further research on the drug is usually abandoned. At the end of phase II we are able to state whether the treatment has any potential benefit in humans, but we can not state that it is as effective or safe as other treatments for that disease. For this reason, we go on to the last phase of evaluation (phase III) in which the new treatment is compared to a standard therapy.

In some cases phase III evaluation is done by comparing the results of a new treatment with results previously achieved using conventional therapy. However, this approach has often mislead us in the past, and now we more often employ a randomized clinical trial in which half of the patients receive the new treatment and the other half the standard therapy. Phase III trials involve many more patients—usually several hundred to a thousand or more—and are much more difficult and expensive to do. While it might seem simple to treat a patient with a new therapy and determine whether he/she feels better, the fact that the patient feels better may not be related to the treatment. This is because even ineffective treatments will often make a patient feel better. This is called the placebo effect. This placebo effect occurs even when the new treatment has quite a few side effects. However, before we routinely use a drug to treat cancer patients, we want to know that it has more than a placebo effect. Just because a drug causes a tumor to shrink, it does not always follow that the drug will relieve pain or other symptoms of cancer.

The same is true for prolonging life. Sometimes it is easy to determine if a drug will cure patients—or at least make them live longer. For example, if a group of patients has an untreatable cancer that is invariably fatal in a short time—e.g. six months—and a new treatment prolongs life so that all (or almost all) patients live at least two years, it is easy to conclude that there is a benefit. Fortunately for patients and unfortunately for science it is not usually that simple, especially for diseases such as breast cancer. No treatment has yet been identified that will cure a breast cancer patient once the disease has spread to distant sites, such as lung, bone, liver, or brain. However, this does not mean the patient will die right away, or even soon. Some patients will live for only a few months after the detection of distant spread. At least half will live for two to three years. And some will live for a decade or more after the disease has spread. A very few have been reported to live with distant metastases for 30 to 40 years! Thus, if a doctor treats a small number of patients—e.g. 20 to 30—and a few of them live for five years, how does he/she know they wouldn't have lived that long without the treatment or with more conventional therapy?

Before a new drug is approved by the FDA, it must go through all three phases of evaluation. Before any patient is enrolled, the trials must be approved by both the FDA and a local human protection committee or institutional review board (IRB). Among the things that the human protection committee evaluates most carefully is the informed consent document to insure that patients who enroll in the study will be told all that is known about the benefits of this drug as well as the potential dangers.

Until the drug is approved by the FDA for general use, however, only those patients who are enrolled in these phase I, phase II, or phase III trials can get the drug. Thus, we have a long-standing tradition in the United States of restricting the right of a physician to prescribe a drug or for a patient to have access to a drug until these studies are completed. We have been proud of the fact that this process has saved the American public from tragedies that occurred in countries with less stringent requirements for drug approval. The most striking example of such a tragedy was thalidamide, a drug used to alleviate the morning sickness associated with pregnancy; many of the children born to women who took this drug were severely deformed.

Once a drug is approved by the FDA, however, we do not generally restrict a physician's right to prescribe a drug even at doses or for conditions that were not originally described in the FDA approval. In addition, restrictions on the use of surgery and other procedures that do not come under the purview of the FDA have, in the past, been left to the discretion of the hospitals where these procedures are performed.

However, In the past 40 years the number of new therapies and technologies developed by the medical profession and the pharmaceutical industry exceed by many fold the number introduced in any prior century of medical history. This has contributed to a rapid escalation in the cost of medical care. In some cases it has also resulted in adding to, rather than alleviating, the suffering of our patients. This happens when a toxic therapy is accepted without adequate evaluation and is subsequently found to have no greater value than standard treatments.

High dose chemotherapy with autologous bone marrow transplant falls under the category of a treatment that does not require FDA approval. All of the drugs used in these high dose regimens have been previously approved for use at lower doses to treat either breast cancer or other type of cancers. Since these drugs are known to be effective at low doses, it would have been very surprising if the phase II studies of high dose chemotherapy with bone marrow transplant had resulted in no tumor shrinkage in any of these patients. The important question—which has not been answered—is: Are the high doses of chemotherapy and bone marrow transplant as good as or better than conventional chemotherapy?

Most experts in the field of breast cancer and bone marrow transplant agree that there is very little or no benefit from the use of this technique in patients whose breast cancer has grown while receiving conventional dose chemotherapy. The most promising results are from studies in which patients have not been given prior chemotherapy to shrink their metastases. (Metastases are the tumor growths that occur throughout the body when breast cancer spreads from its original site in the breast). In most of the published studies, patients were first given four to six months of conventional dose chemotherapy; if their tumor shrank as a result of the conventional dose treatment, they were then immediately given one or two additional courses of high dose chemotherapy with bone marrow transplant. In these trials, the percentage of patients whose tumor disappeared completely after this treatment was considerably higher than that reported in previous years using conventional dose chemotherapy. However, the percentage of patients in these transplant studies whose tumor completely disappeared before the high dose chemotherapy was given was also much higher than previously reported from studies using the same conventional dose chemotherapy. This suggests that the patients enrolled in these transplant studies were in some way different from the patients enrolled in other trials. It is likely that their disease was more responsive to chemotherapy.

Only 6 or 7 of these trials have published results on the survival of patients with metastatic (or wide spread) breast cancer treated with high dose chemotherapy and bone marrow transplant. In these studies the average (or median) survival of the transplanted patients was not longer and might even be slightly shorter than than of patients treated with conventional chemotherapy. Similarly, the percentage of patients alive at two to five years following transplant was no greater than that achieved with the best conventional chemotherapy regimens. There is absolutely no evidence that any woman has been cured with high dose chemotherapy and bone marrow transplant who would not have been cured with conventional therapy.

Several phase II studies have now been published on the potential benefits of high dose chemotherapy and bone marrow transplant in women whose cancer has not yet spread widely (i.e. metastasized to distant organs). These studies using high dose chemotherapy and bone marrow transplant as an adjuvant in patients with 10 or more positive nodes suggest that the high dose chemotherapy may prolong the time until the cancer comes back in distant organs. None of these studies has shown that this treatment will prolong the lives of these patients. As with the use of this treatment in patients with wide spread disease, there is not yet evidence that any of these patients have been cured with this therapy.

Tumor seems to disappear more completely following high dose chemotherapy and bone marrow transplant than following conventional therapy. At the same time, there is no evidence that this treatment prolongs patient survival. In the face of this uncertainty about whether there really is a net benefit for using high dose chemotherapy and bone marrow transplant in any group of breast cancer patients, we have initiated three nation-wide randomized trials to evaluate this therapy. Almost all American leaders in the study of breast cancer have publicly endorsed these studies. Most of the prestigious medical Institutions of this country have enrolled patients on these studies, including Duke University, Johns Hopkins University, the Dana-Farber Cancer Institute at Harvard, the University of Pennsylvania, the University of Chicago, the University of Colorado, and the University of California, San Francisco. (This is only a partial list.) It would be unethical to run these trials if it were already known that high dose chemotherapy and bone marrow transplant were better than conventional chemotherapy.

Randomized trials frequently show that a treatment thought to be promising in early trials is not as good as we have hoped. In the treatment of breast cancer we have a very good example: the radical mastectomy. This form of surgery, which removes the breast, all the muscles on the chest wall, skin overlying these muscles (thus requiring a skin graft) and many lymph nodes was our standard treatment for breast cancer during the first 70 years of this century. This form of surgery was more mutilating than the surgery used either today or in the 19th century. It was also more expensive, since it required that the patient be in the operating room for longer period of time; the surgeon had to be very skilled, and it took weeks for the patient to recover from the operation. Eventually we were able to show in randomized trials that this surgery was not associated with a longer life and did not cure more patients than less mutilating and less expensive surgical procedures. But this was only after 5–7 million women had received the operation.

Like the radical mastectomy, high dose chemotherapy and bone marrow transplant "makes sense" to the average person. It is a powerful and technologically demanding approach to a problem that is difficult to understand and that strikes fear in the heart of every woman. It is a big solution to a big problem! For this reason, it is difficult for most patients to understand why they can only receive this treatment if they are in a trial. The orderly process of performing phase I, II, and III studies takes years. Most women with breast cancer do not feel they can wait that long. They frequently see this treatment as their only hope.

After years of practicing medicine, I am convinced that the single most important element contributing to a good quality of life is hope. Take away hope, and even the cured patient will suffer for the remainder of her life. But hope is not generated by facts and figures. It is the province of healers, whether the healer is a physician, a nurse, a priest, or a provider of a remedy outside the mainstream of medicine. Thus if anyone, including those who know very little about the subject, says to a patient—"Your only hope for cure is high dose chemotherapy and a bone marrow transplant"—it is likely to haunt the patient until she has acted on this recommendation. While making treatment decisions, breast cancer patients are extremely vulnerable. They want to make sure they have not overlooked a single opportunity. And the media plays on this vulnerability. The results of relatively minor laboratory experiments are reported in our daily newspapers without a clear indication that such experiments are (a) not likely to effect the treatment of any human disease and (b) if they do lead to an effective treatment, it is not likely to be available for years or even decades. Once instilled in a patient's heart, how can any of us take away that which the patient has concluded—correctly or incorrectly—is her only hope?

In this charged atmosphere it has been difficult for Insurors to develop a policy regarding payment for high dose chemotherapy and bone marrow transplant for breast cancer. Those who pay for health insurance—most often businesses and governments—demand that escalating health care costs be controlled. One rational way to cut costs is to stop paying for therapies that are not effective, and many insurance companies now require rigorous evidence that a treatment is truly safe and effective before paying for it, much as the FDA does before approving a new drug. When high does chemotherapy and bone marrow transplant is assessed in this way, most insurors have found that there are insufficient data to justify paying for this as standard treatment.

High dose chemotherapy and bone marrow transplant is a toxic and very costly treatment.[1] Those who have concluded that this is the single best hope for a cure find it difficult not to feel that cost is a principle motivation of the insuror who denies coverage.

Traditionally, insurance contracts have excluded payment for experimental treatments. However, if the insuror does not pay for the medical costs of the patients who are in these trials, the trials will never be completed. Doctors who passionately believe in this treatment argue that high does chemotherapy and bone marrow transplant is not experimental, hoping that insurors will then allow them to either prescribe the therapy or at least evaluate it further.[2] In recent years several insurors, including some Blue Cross and Blue Shield plans, have sought to alleviate this problem by raising special funds to pay for the costs of their patients when they are enrolled in trials supported by the National Cancer Institute even if they don't pay for the cost of this treatment outside of such trials.

How do we resolve this conflict between the humanistic desire to comfort the seriously ill and the scientific need to find out which treatments really work? I am convinced it is NOT by abandoning rigorous assessment of new treatments. To do so will not only increase the cost of medicine, it will lead us down many blind alleys.

---

[1] This therapy was (and is) much more expensive than conventional therapy. Usually prolonged hospitalization is necessary with multiple transfusions of blood and blood products, the administration of expensive antibiotics, and the use of isolation procedures to protect the patients from infection. In the early days a course of treatment averaged more than $150,000. However, as often happens when a new treatment is developed, the average price has fallen considerable, and the current average prices are now more often in the $60,000 to $90,000 range. None-the-less, this high price tag for the treatment of a common disease, such as breast cancer, represents a substantial cost to insurors. At the same time, it is a source of potential profit for hospitals, since this treatment fills beds now empty as the average stay for the treatment of other types of disease has fallen dramatically. Although very few doctors have thus far made much personal wealth from the administration of high dose chemotherapy and bone marrow transplantation, many hospitals, especially university hospitals, and anxious to hire physicians with expertise in administering this therapy, and even physician jobs are unusually secure in the midst of the current era of constraint.

[2] This argument is: High dose chemotherapy and bone marrow transplant causes tumors to shrink, just as conventional therapy does. There is no evidence that the lives of these patients are shortened by this process. Therefore, it is an effective therapy even if we do not know if it is more or less effective than conventional therapy.

In some cases—like that of the radical mastectomy—it may delay our search for better therapies for decades or even centuries. Instead we need to pay for the treatment of any patient who participates in national clinical trials and speed up the process of evaluation so there is not such a long delay between the promise and the reality of a new therapy.

Recent experiences of AIDS activists illustrate the importance of completing proper (usually randomized) trials before making a therapy generally available. A decade ago, when AIDS activists first began to demand that drugs be available to patients before trials were completed, accrual to some studies decreased substantially. This seemed to slow the process of finding a cure. However, I recently participated in a meeting to assess data for a new drug to treat an AIDS related tumor. Several AIDS activists participated in this meeting, and I was impressed with how carefully and critically they examined the data. This was a contrast to what I had seen 10 years earlier. During a break I asked them how they have arrived at this point. They answered: "Watching thousands of our friends die in spite of our best effort lead us to realize that there were more to this than just making the treatments available."

The Blue Cross and Blue Shield Association (BCBSA) welcomes this opportunity to provide written testimony to the Subcommittee on the important issue of coverage for high dose chemotherapy with autologous bone marrow (or stem cell) transplant (HDC/ABMT) in the treatment of breast cancer. These comments will begin with brief background information about the Blue Cross and Blue Shield Association and its technology assessment function. It will then address the scientific evidence concerning the efficacy of HDC/ABMT for breast cancer and the clinical controversy generated by the lack of adequate evidence. Finally, I will describe the BCBSA Demonstration Project on Breast Cancer Treatment, an innovative effort to resolve this controversy. Federal employees have access to the Demonstration Project through the Blue Cross and Blue Shield Federal Employee Program (FEP) and six other FEHB plans that have chosen to participate in the Demonstration Project.

The BCBSA believes that support of essential clinical trails of HDC/ABMT rather than coverage in all settings is the only option third-party payers have if they wish to promote the rational use of this new treatment modality. Coverage without demonstrated efficacy will facilitate broad dissemination of a toxic and costly treatment with no known clinical benefit.

BACKGROUND ON THE BCBSA AND TECHNOLOGY EVALUATION CENTER (TEC)

The BCBSA is the national coordinating agency for the 69 independent, locally governed Blue Cross and Blue Shield Plans. The BCBSA serves as the cohesive force that brings these autonomous, non-profit Plans together into a national system. As a system, we are the nation's largest and oldest provider of health care coverage, currently covering 67 million members or more than one in four Americans. Our Plans operate 92 health maintenance organizations (HMOs) and 56 Preferred Provider Organizations (PPOs) nationwide. Four and one-half million federal employees and their dependents have their health care coverage through the Blue Cross and Blue Shield Federal Employees Program (FEP).

The BCBSA provides many support services to Blue Cross and Blue Shield Plans and FEP. Technology assessment through the BCBSA Technology Evaluation Center (TEC) is one of these services.

TEC is one of the nations leading technology evaluation efforts, having conducted more than 200 assessments since its creation in 1984. TEC has been a pioneer in the use of scientific evidence to determine the safety and efficacy of new medical technologies. The TEC assessments are scientific opinions meant to provide information to those who deliver and manage medical care.

In September of 1993, the TEC program expanded to other payers with the collaboration of Kaiser Permanente. David Eddy, M.D., Ph.D., senior advisor for health policy and management for Kaiser, concurrently assumed the role of the program's Chief Scientific Advisor. The Medical Advisory Panel, which is the program's external review team, was expanded to include prominent experts in scientific methods, clinical research, and medical practice. A majority of the panel's members are now independent medical experts with no affiliation with health care payers. Assessments are now available to all interested parties on a subscription basis.

The TEC Program uses five criteria to determine whether the technology in question improves health outcomes such as length of life, ability to function, or quality of life. Cost is not a consideration in technology evaluation. The five TEC criteria are:

1. The technology must have final approval from the appropriate government regulatory bodies.

2. The scientific evidence must permit conclusions concerning the effect of the technology on health outcomes.

3. The technology must improve the net health outcome.

4. The technology must be as beneficial as any established alternatives.

5. The improvement must be attainable outside the investigational settings.

Many BCBSA Plans will consider only technologies that meet all five TEC criteria to be eligible for coverage. These Plans find new medical technologies that do not meet all the criteria to be investigational.

THE EFFICACY OF HDC/ABMT FOR BREAST CANCER

A major issue for insurers is the demand for coverage of a technology before there are data demonstrating its efficacy. One such treatment, HDC/ABMT for breast cancer, has been the source of much controversy. Clinical studies of HDC/ABMT conducted to date have not established that this treatment is as safe and effective as conventional chemotherapy in the treatment of advanced and early but high-risk breast cancer. Many BCBS Plans exclude coverage for the treatment because they consider it to be investigational. HDC/ABMT for breast cancer has been evaluated three times by the Association's Medical Advisory Panel in recent years: in 1988, in 1991 by David Eddy, M.D., Ph.D., and most recently, on July 28, 1994.

HDC/ABMT for breast cancer does not meet the five TEC criteria. There has been an absence of well-controlled trials, existing clinical series are poorly matched, and small differences in survival demonstrated between HDC/ABMT and conventional chemotherapy for breast cancer to date have not been statistically significant. Furthermore, treatment-related mortality and morbidity from HDC/ABMT exceed that from conventional chemotherapy.

Other technology assessment bodies agree with the conclusions of TEC. Medicare does not provide coverage for HDC/ABMT for breast cancer or any other solid tumor. The AMA technology assessment program, DATTA, surveyed expert physicians on the reference panel on the safety and effectiveness of HDC/ABMT for breast cancer in 1991. In every instance queried, the panel "considered high dose chemotherapy for breast cancer to be investigational in terms of both its safety and effectiveness." "No panelist considered the therapy established in terms of its safety or effectiveness while at least one panelist considered it unacceptable for each of the given clinical situations."

ECRI, a proprietary technology assessment and information service, completed an assessment of HDC/ABMT for breast cancer in June of 1994. ECRI concluded that the treatment "is diffusing into the health care system before there is any clear evidence that the treatment is better than conventional therapies." Nearly two-thirds of high dose chemotherapy with stem cell rescue regimens yielded shorter response durations than conventional chemotherapy. And most high dose chemotherapy with stem cell rescue regimens are associated with shorter survival times compared to conventional regimens, ECRI found.

Onocology research experts believe that HDC/ABMT should only be available in well-designed clinical trials that will help determine the efficacy of the treatment. The National Cancer Institute (NCI) has taken the position that clinical trials are needed to determine the safety and efficacy of HDC/ABMT for breast cancer prior to wide spread dissemination of the treatment. "Currently, NCI sponsored clinical trials are carefully addressing this important issue, because for patients with solid tumors, more data are needed to definitely establish the role of ABMT as standard treatment in these disease settings. Although it is not within the mandate of the NCI to determine insurance coverage policy, we believe it is scientifically, financially and clinically necessary that formal scientific demonstration of ABMT benefit occur prior to the unlimited dissemination of such a toxic and expensive therapy." The BCBSA and OPM are supporting the NCI trials through the Demonstration Project on Breast Cancer Treatment, described below.

In 1993, a consensus conference in Lyon, France, concluded that there was "insufficient evidence to justify the use of HDC/ABMT outside the setting of a clinical trial for any stage of breast cancer." This position was reiterated by Dr. Karen Antman, current president of the American Society for Clinical Oncology (ASCO) during ASCO's 1994 annual meeting.

DEMONSTRATION PROJECT ON BREAST CANCER TREATMENT

Despite the lack of conclusive evidence that HDC/ABMT is as good as, worse, or better than conventional chemotherapy for breast cancer, coverage denials by BCBS Plans and other payers have generated unprecedented media interest and litigation.

Some researchers advocate the treatment and women have sued, convinced that this treatment is their last hope. Some subscribers want access to this service regardless of the lack of scientific evidence supporting efficacy. Unfortunately, as an editorial in the Journal of the National Cancer Institute stated, some members of the oncology community "have raised the public's expectation far above what is supported by the published data. We have no evidence as of yet that any patient will be cured by this therapy who would not have been cured by more conventional treatment" (Henderson, 1991).

The Demonstration Project on Breast Cancer Treatment is an innovative effort to help resolve the clinical controversy surrounding the efficacy of HDC/ABMT for breast cancer. The Demonstration Project is an attempt to return the debate to the appropriate forum of clinical research and away from the courtroom and television. Only well-designed research can answer the question "does HDC/ABMT work for breast cancer."

The purpose of the Demonstration Project is to support randomized controlled clinical trials comparing the efficacy of HDC/ABMT with that of conventional chemotherapy in the treatment of advanced breast cancer and early breast cancer with poor prognosis. The clinical trials are being sponsored by the National Cancer Institute (NCI), the Clinical Trials Cooperative Groups, and the Philadelphia Bone Marrow Transplant Group. It is hoped that increased financial support for this costly investigational treatment will speed accruals to the trials while providing our subscribers with access to this treatment. The Demonstration Project is supporting two multicenter randomized trials for women with State II/III breast cancer and 10 or more positive nodes (designated CALGB 9082 an INT 0121 by the NCI) and one multicenter randomized trial for women with Stage IV metastatic disease (the Philadelphia Protocol, PBT–1).

The Demonstration Project provides financial support, on behalf of BCBS members, to institutions that are participating in the trials and have entered into contracts with the BCBSA. The all-inclusive financial support payments are separate and distinct from coverage. They constitute support for clinical research and not benefit payments. The financial support payments defray a significant portion of the patient care costs of HDC/ABMT, including impatient, physician and ancillary services. Participating institutions are expected to share in the costs of treatment as well.

Currently, 15 Blue Cross and Blue Shield Plans and the Federal Employee Program, accounting for 40 percent of our membership, are participating in the Demonstration Project. The office of Personnel Management and the BCBSA opened the Demonstration Project to non-Blue FEHB Plans in 1992. Six FEHB Plans, in addition to the Blue Cross and Blue Shield FEP program, has chosen to participate in the program. To date, 43 hospitals are participating, and eligible hospitals are welcome to enter into contracts at any time. Several of the supported trials are accruing very well and we believe our support contributes to the rapid accrual. One trail has surpassed its accrual goal and is continuing to enter patients to increase its power.

BCBS Plans and the Office of Personnel Management for the Federal Employee Health Benefit Plans have been willing to invest resources in the Demonstration Project to obtain the clinical data necessary for determining the efficacy of this toxic and costly treatment. In the absence of such financial support, the trials might not be conducted or completed. These well-designed, large, randomized multicenter trials will provide the date essential for assessing this technology. Prior studies have been inadequate. During this period when efficacy is being evaluated, the Demonstration Project provides access to the treatment through trials for eligible women who are desperate to try any promising therapy.

The BCBSA believes strongly that support of well-designed clinical trials is the only responsible course third-party payers can follow at this time to resolve the controversy over coverage for HDC/ABMT. In the past, the Demonstration Project has limited its support to the Phase III national randomized trials. A new Clinical Trial Support Program initiated in July of 1994 will support additional trials. We are convening a national advisory committee to help us select well-designed trials that can yield definitive data on important scientific questions.

Ms. NORTON. Thank you very much, Dr. Henderson.

Dr. Jones.

Dr. JONES. I am Dr. Roy Jones.

Ms. NORTON. Dr. Jones, may I say for the record, would you and the next witness summarize your testimony and submit the full testimony for the record?

Dr. JONES. Yes, I will. I am Dr. Roy Jones, Director of the Bone Marrow Transplant Program at the University of Colorado. High dose chemotherapy and bone marrow transplant has emerged as the most potent, if not the most potent treatment, for advanced or high risk breast cancer. Thousands of patients have received them.

Recently, Dr. Bill Peters of Duke University summarized the results from more than 1,000 patients treated with BMT for metastatic breast cancer and 900 patients treated for primary high risk primary breast cancer followed for five years or more. The results tend to show the patients with metastatic breast cancer have five-year tumor free survival of 15 to 20 percent for breast cancer patients above the results of standard conventional chemotherapy. The five-year relapse-free survival for high risk primary breast cancer treated with BMT is 35 percent better than any result reported in medical literature by any research group using any conventional treatment. I agree with the NCI staff and OPM, and Dr. Henderson that coin-flip trials are required to definitively prove the superiority of these treatments. But available evidence from 8 to 10 years of these tests is clear: these programs are very effective.

While awaiting the coin-flip trial results, breast cancer has now become the single disease most commonly treated with bone marrow transplant in the United States. During this period a number of other programs outside these coin-flip trials have been designed at research centers.

The present OPM policies recommends denial for reimbursement of this treatment or approves coverage only for patients participating in coin-flip trials. That is, the patient and their doctor in these trials cannot select bone marrow transplant if they preferred. Most indemnity insurers such as Prudential, Aetna, Mutual of Omaha, and many regional Blue Cross–Blue Shield plans approve reimbursement for breast cancer BMT outside of this requirement.

The OPM policy compels patients to enroll in two specific types of research programs to gain access to treatment, both of them coin flips. Other research and treatment programs such as those conducted at most of the major cancer centers described here allow access to additional programs outside of the coin-flip requirement. OPM justifies their policy by noting that until the coin-flip trials are fully completed and analyzed, definitive proof for the benefits of BMT are lacking.

It is important for you to know that proof of efficacy through coin-flip trials is specifically lacking for each and every disease for which OPM presently reimburses for bone marrow transplant. Further, they reimburse for cancer situations in cases where we are quite well convinced the efficacy is less than any demonstrable benefit for breast cancer at this time. Thus, reimbursement in these circumstances seems likely, at least to me, to be arbitrary, irrational, capricious and discriminatory. Most medical and surgical treatments have never been fully demonstrated to have proof of effectiveness based upon coin-flip trials. If reimbursement were systematically denied for each and every medical treatment for which there is coin-flip proof of superiority, your health care crisis would be solved because health care reimbursements would decline by more than 50 to 75 percent.

I do not advocate unrestricted reimbursement for bone marrow transplant outside of the research setting. Until this technology is optimized for cost-effectiveness and efficacy, its administration should be restricted to research centers with a proven track record of research productivity. Otherwise, halfway technology will be given to patients at the price of reduced benefit and increased cost.

Neither the insurance industry nor any arm of the Federal Government has accepted more than limited responsibility to pay for patient care costs of therapies like BMT. That is OPM and the National Cancer Institute today would not pay the patient care costs of investigation of BMT studies in ovarian cancer, an area of promising new research in the opinion of many investigators.

How are these studies done today? How were they done in the past so we could reach the coin-flip trial stage? Only through a few generous insurers, from insurance mistakes, wealthy patients capable of paying out of pocket, and litigation. The NCI pays for the research costs of these efforts, namely computers, data clerks, drugs, and so forth but does not pay for routine patient care costs such as nurses, blood tests, x-rays and so forth. The equation is quite simple: If there is no patient care reimbursement, there is no BMT research, there are no coin-flip studies which derive from them, and there are no improved treatments for cancer.

Therefore, how should OPM respond to the demands for reimbursement for new high technology treatment? In the case of breast cancer, evidence from the medical literature, breast cancer experts and the courts seems clear: their policy should change.

Importantly, how should the next reimbursement challenge be handled and how should health care reform address this issue?

I suggest that new high technology treatments for cancer should be reimbursed if they are approved by the NCI, its cooperative groups or designated cancer centers. These treatments should be administered at centers of excellence approved by these groups and centers that have proven track records of research productivity and qualification. Such centers are widely dispersed throughout the country and, therefore, guarantee reasonable access for any patient who wants to get into these particular trials. This coverage must be mandated for any insurer, including managed care plans and, importantly, self-ensuring companies which would be a problem based on the ERISA statute. Only after cost-effectiveness, not just effectiveness, is stable and optimized would these therapies be disseminated to the community.

How can we justify this kind of reimbursement requirement? If we have no policy, the future will see further erosion of access to and the developments of new treatments with disproportionate effects on lower income patients. The NCI already subsidizes the research costs. If all categories of insurers do not participate in reimbursing for these treatments, why should they benefit from any cost savings these treatments produce?

Federal employees deserve access to the finest in medical treatment. Based on standards set by most indemnity insurers, standards of evaluation used by OPM to approve other marrow transplant procedures, and results available in medical literature, marrow transplant for breast cancer should be a medical benefit when performed in centers of excellence. Reimbursement should not be restricted to a few coin-flip trials no matter how meritorious they are designed.

Eagerness to complete these trials does not justify coercion to enroll in research studies where half the patients may be forced to take a treatment they don't want. Access to the full range of NCI-approved trials removes coercion and optimizes patient access to treatments they and their doctors want, limits the dissemination of incompletely-studied high technology, guarantees insurer participation in treatments from which they can benefit, and optimizes rapid translation of promising new treatments to patients with otherwise fatal diseases.

Please require OPM to require reimbursement for these programs.

Thank you.

[The prepared statement of Dr. Jones follows:]

PREPARED STATEMENT OF DR. ROY B. JONES, DIRECTOR OF THE BONE MARROW TRANSPLANT PROGRAM, UNIVERSITY OF COLORADO

Madam Chairman, Ladies and Gentlemen: I am Director of Bone Marrow Transplant Program at the University of Colorado. I have been an investigator and treating physician in the field of marrow transplantion or BMT for breast cancer since research began in this area. Thank you for the opportunity to testify.

High-Dose Chemotherapy and BMT has emerged as the most potent treatment yet developed for advanced or high-risk breast cancer. Thousands of patients have been treated with these programs. Recently Dr. Bill Peters of Duke has collated data from more than 1000 patients treated with BMT for metastitic breast cancer and more than 900 patients treated for high-risk primary breast cancer, both groups followed for more than 5 years. Patients with metastic breast cancer have a 5-year tumor-free survival 15–20% above results when conventional therapy was given at three of America's most prestigious cancer hospitals. The 5-year relapse-free survival for high-risk primary breast cancer treated with BMT is 35% better than the any result reported in the medical literature by any research group using any conventional treatment. I agree with NCI staff and OPM that coinflip trials are required to definitively prove the superiority of these treatments, but available evidence from 8–10 years of research is clear. These programs are very effective.

While awaiting the coinflip trail results, breast cancer has ow become the disease most frequently treated with BMT in the United States. During this period, many other research programs approved and subsidized by the National Cancer Institute and their regional cancer cancers seek to improve the curative potential of marrow transplantation, reduce its cost and risk, and introduce new drugs and other types of treatments to marrow transplant regimens.

Present OPM policy recommends denial of reimbursement for this treatment or approves coverage only for patients participating in two coinflip trails which assign treatment to either BMT or conventional therapy by change. That is, the patient and their doctor cannot select BMT if they prefer it. Most indemnity insurers such as Prudential, Aetna, Metropolitan, Mutual of Omaha, and many regional Blue Cross/Blue Shield indemnity plans approve reimbursement for breast cancer BMT without this requirement.

This policy compels patients to enroll in two specific research program to gain access to treatment. Other research and treatment programs approved and subsidized by the NCI permit access to BMT without a coinflip and should be available to patients as alternatives. Failure to allow access to these options is coercive.

OPM justifies its policy by noting that, until the coinflip trails are completed and analyzed, definitive proof of BMT superiority is lacking. It is important to point out that randomized trails are specifically lacking for each and every disease for which BMT is reimbursed now. In fact, breast cancer researchers may be the first to complete such trails. Further, many cancer situations which routinely receive BMT approval by OMP have results which are unequivocally inferior to those for breast cancer. OPM is using a standard never before applied in this area to decline reimbursement for breast cancer BMT. Thus, reimbursement for these situations and not for breast cancer is arbitrary, irrational, capricious, and discriminatory. Most medical and surgical treatments have never been proven superior by coinflip trails, but are administered based upon physicians best judgment from extensive non-coinflip data.

If reimbursement were systematically denied for each treatment lacking coinflip proof of superiority or for which medical researchers have concluded that further research is indicated, the financial crisis in health care would solved—payments would drop by at least 50–75%.

I do not advocate unrestricted reimbursement for BMT for breast cancer outside the research setting. Until this technology is optimized for cost-effectiveness, its administration should be restricted to research centers with proven research productivity. Otherwise, half-way technology is given to patients at the price of reduced benefit and increased cost.

Neither the insurance industry nor any arm of the federal government has accepted more than limited responsibility to pay for the patient care cost of newer therapies like BMT. That is, OPM and the National Cancer Institute would today not pay for patient care costs for investigation of BMT studies for ovarian cancer, a promising new area of research. How are these studies and were the earlier breast cancer studies performed? Only through a few generous insurers, frank insurance mistakes, wealthy patients who can pay out of pocket, and litigation. The NCI pays for research costs of these efforts—such as computers, data clerks, and drugs, but not for routine patient care costs—such as nurses, blood tests, x/rays and so forth. The equation is simple—if there is not patient care reimbursement, there is no BMT research, no coin-flip studies which derive from them, and no improved treatments for cancer.

How should OPM respond to reimbursement demands for new, high-technology treatments? In the case of breast cancer, evidence from the medical literature, breast cancer experts, and the courts is clear. Their policy should change. But importantly, how should the next reimbursement challenge be handled, and how should health care reform address this issue?

I suggest that new high-technology treatments for cancer should be reimbursed if they are approved by the NCI, its cooperative groups, or its designated cancer centers. These treatments should only be administered at centers of excellence, approved by these groups, which have proven track records of treatment results and research excellence. Such centers are widely dispersed throughout the country and guarantee access for any patient wishing treatment. This coverage must be mandated for any insurer, including managed care plans and self insuring companies. Only after cost-effectiveness, not just effectiveness, is stable and optimized would these therapies be disseminated to the community.

How can we justify reimbursement requirements? If we have no policy, the future will see further erosion of access to and development of these treatments, with disproportionate effects on lower income patients. The NCI already subsidizes the research costs of these trails. If all categories of insurers do not participate in reimbursing for these treatments, why should they be allowed to benefit from any cost savings produced by treatment advances?

Federal employees deserve access to the finest medical treatment. Based on standards set by most indemnity insurers, standards of evaluation used by OPM to approve other marrow transplant procedures, and results available in the medical literature, marrow transplant for breast cancer should be a covered benefit when performed in centers of excellence conducting peer-reviewed research studies. Reimbursement should not be restricted to a few coin-flip trails no matter how meritorious their design. Eagerness to complete these trails does not justify coercion to enroll in research studies where half the patients must take a treatment they may not want. Access to the full range of NCI-approved trials removes coercion and optimizes patient access to treatments they and their doctors want, limits the dissemination of incompletely studied high technology, guarantees insurer participation in treatments from which they can benefit, and optimizes rapid translation of promising new treatments to patients with otherwise fatal diseases. Please require OPM to approve reimbursement for these programs.

Thank you very much.

[Addendum Materials]

UNIVERSITY OF COLORADO HEALTH SCIENCES CENTER,
Denver, CO, June 6, 1994.

Re Bone marrow transplant procedures for breast cancer.

Hon. JAMES KING,
Director, Office of Personnel Management,
Washington, DC.

DEAR MR. KING: We are writing to encourage the Office of Personnel Management to revise its present position that bone marrow transplant procedures for breast cancer are "experimental or investigational" and are not subject to reimbursement by government sponsored or directed health plans. We believe that there are three basic grounds to suggest that this judgment is outdated and should be revised:

1. OUTCOME DATA FROM THE PROCEDURE

There is now 7–10 years of follow-up data from many hundreds of patients with metastatic tumors who have received this treatment at the most prestigious cancer treatment institutions in the United States. The consensus from at least five different centers (Duke University, Dana Farber Cancer Institute, Harvard Medical School, The MD Anderson Hospital, and the University of Chicago) have suggested that between 15–30% patients treated experience greater than five year relapse-free survival.

The largest series in the medical literature for patients with metastatic breast cancer receiving conventional chemotherapy suggests that anywhere from 0.3% to 2% of patients would be expected to achieve a similar status (The Mayo Clinic, MD Anderson Hospital, Roswell Park Memorial Institute). This data suggests superior outcome for patients treated with bone marrow transplant compared to those treated with conventional therapy. A nationwide randomized trial is presently underway to confirm this outcome.

In patients with Stage II or Stage III breast cancer and more than 10 involved axillary lymph nodes, the data are striking. More than 500 patients have been treated with lead follow-up in excess of five years and median follow-up in the three to four year range. At this time 70–80% of patients remain alive and free of tumor compared to an anticipated 25–40% of patients remaining alive and free of tumor from a broad variety of standard chemotherapy studies. These results are being evaluated in nationwide randomized trials as well.

2. LEGAL AND MEDICAL DEFINITIONS OF "INVESTIGATIONAL OR EXPERIMENTAL" APPLICABLE TO INSURANCE REIMBURSEMENT

Definitions of investigational or experimental vary widely, but usually coalesce about the concept that there is insufficient data to demonstrate efficacy and safety of a procedure. Others choose to define these terms as applicable until randomized control trials of the newer treatment versus conventional treatment are carried out and demonstrate superiority of outcome.

There can be little doubt that the efficacy of bone marrow transplant procedures for breast cancer has been demonstrated. The data cited above, and the explosive growth of the use of this procedure in the United States, all suggest that a broad consensus of physicians recognize this efficacy. There are now large numbers of legal precedents available to suggest that courts have not accepted the claim that this procedure is experimental or investigational. The vast majority of court decisions in this area support the concept that this procedure is neither experimental nor investigational in any reasonable definition of those terms.

Requiring that a procedure is defined as experimental or investigational until its superiority is proved by randomized control trials is a procedure that has never been used by physicians, insurers, or government agencies. The expense and difficulty of these trials dictate that a high percentage of medical treatments have never undergone them. Furthermore, the efficacy of many treatments is obvious enough that it seems appropriate to physicians to apply them without the "gold standard of proof." While we heartily support the use of randomized trials to confirm the superiority of these bone marrow transplant procedures over conventional therapy, we do not believe that the "silver standard of evidence" available now from the literature should be ignored. The evidence to support the efficacy of these procedures is far in excess of many commonly used and reimbursed medical treatments.

3. CONSISTENCY OF REIMBURSEMENT POLICY

Finally, government supported insurance plans reimburse for a number of indications for bone marrow transplantation that are far more speculative in terms of efficacy or cost fluctuation.

For example, data supporting the use of bone marrow transplantation in childhood neuroblastoma or in female germ cell tumor of the ovaries is far less extensive than that supporting breast cancer. There is a broad consensus in the literature that bone marrow transplant for chemotherapy-insensitive lymphoma is much less efficacious than transplant for breast cancer. All of these procedures are routinely reimbursed under Medicare guidelines. Over the past year, five states have either mandated reimbursement for breast cancer or mandated that insurance companies make available policies which will reimburse for marrow transplants for breast cancer on an elective basis.

In conclusion, we hope that the Office of Personnel Management will reconsider its policy decision in this matter. In particular, we hope that the Office of Personnel Management will mandate reimbursement for trials of high-dose chemotherapy endorsed by the National Cancer Institute or its comprehensive cancer centers. Failure to support these efforts runs counter to recommendations of the National Cancer Institute, the government agency with the greatest expertise in this area.

Thank you very much for your consideration of these matters.

> Sincerely,
>> Roy B. Jones, M.D., Ph. D., Director, Bone Marrow Transplant Program, University of Colorado, Denver, CO; William P. Peters, M.D., Ph. D., Director, Bone Marrow Transplant Program, Duke University Medical Center, Durham, NC; Stephanie F. Williams, M.D., Co-Director, Bone Marrow Transplant Program, University of Chicago, Chicago, IL; Gary Spitzer, M.D., Professor of Medicine, St. Louis University Medical Center, St. Louis, MO; Richard Champlin, M.D., MD Anderson Cancer Center, Houston, TX; Nancy Davidson, M.D., Johns Hopkins Oncology Center, Baltimore, MD.

U.S. OFFICE OF PERSONNEL MANAGEMENT,
Washington, DC, July 7, 1994.

ROY B. JONES, M.D., Ph.D.,
Director, Bone Morrow Transplant Program, University of Colorado, Denver, CO.

DEAR DR. JONES: Thank you for your letter of June 6, 1994, concerning coverage for high-dose chemotherapy with autologous bone marrow transplantation (HDC/ABMT) for the treatment of breast cancer under the Federal Employees Health Benefits (FEHB) Program.

Our basic responsibility as administrator of the FEHB Program is to make comprehensive, affordable health benefits coverage available to all Federal employees and annuitants, and their family members. All health insurance plans participating in the FEHB Program provide benefits for the treatment of cancer, including breast cancer. However, not all methods of treatment for this condition are covered under all plans.

We are concerned that our carriers should cover treatments that have been demonstrated to be safe and effective. Simply stated, the reason HDC/AMBT is covered for some conditions but not for breast cancer is that the treatment has not yet been shown to be more effective than conventional treatment for this particular disease. We know, however, that it carriers a much higher degree of risk. Mandating coverage for such treatment is not a matter of cost; it's a matter of assuring that the treatments help more than they harm. This is precisely the question that the ongoing clinical trials are addressing.

The Duke University study referenced in your letter states that due to its toxicity, cost, and complexity, at present this treatment should only be offered at major centers of excellence in which patients are entered into randomized comparative trials whenever possible. The conclusion of the study is that evaluation in randomized clinical trials is warranted and currently underway. It does not recommend that HDC/ABMT for breast cancer be considered accepted medical practice or mainstreamed into conventional medicine. Based on this and other medical evidence that we have reviewed, we continue to believe that HDC/ABMT for the treatment of breast cancer is dangerous and its effectiveness unproven. The National Cancer Institute (NCI) has also advised us that HDC/ABMT for breast cancer should not be performed outside the clinical trials setting.

The continuing clinical trials of the use of HDC/ABMT in the treatment of breast cancer serve to define this mode of treatment as investigational for this condition. In negotiating benefits with health insurance plans participating in the FEHB Program, we have not felt it would be in the best interests of our enrollees to require plans to provide coverage for services that fall within this definition. Although we have accepted proposals by several individual FEHB plans to provide coverage for this treatment under certain limited circumstances when determined by plan doctors to be medically necessary and appropriate, we cannot, and do not, require FEHB plans to cover an investigational treatment.

However, we and a number a FEHB plans, including the Government-wide Service Benefit Plan and several of the largest open fee-for-service plans, are participating in a demonstration project to offer Federal members the opportunity to participate in NCI-sponsored clinical trials studying HDC/ABMT for breast cancer in centers of excellence throughout the country, and reimbursement for the associated costs. These trials, which are examining several different NCI-approved protocols, should provide an independent and, we hope, conclusive assessment of the efficacy of HDC/ABMT in the treatment of breast cancer.

Through our participation in this demonstration project, the FEHB Program can contribute to the effort to define the benefits of this treatment for patients with breast cancer. As the Duke University study recommends, we are awaiting the NCI trials results. We will not hesitate to modify our coverage requirements as soon as reliable clinical evidence indicates that HDC/ABMT is at least as effective as conventional treatment for breast cancer and is worth the added risk.

Thank you for the opportunity to respond to you and your colleagues on this issue of mutual concern.

Sincerely,

JAMES B. KING,
Director.

DISSEMINATION AND COMMERCIALIZATION OF HEMATOPOIETIC PROGENITOR CELL TRANSPLANTATION

(By Roy B. Jones and Elizabeth J. Shpall)

Bone Marrow Transplantation (BMT), now including marrow or peripheral blood progenitor cell support following intensive anticancer therapy, has been employed with increasing frequency over the last 10 years. Data from many studies demonstrate that the anticancer effect of dose intensity and graft vs. tumor immunity represent fundamentally important advances in cancer treatment. Large numbers of research studies are presently underway to maximize the therapeutic benefit and cost-effectiveness of these observations.

In recent years, these advances have been accompanied by disturbing developments. Often irrational U.S. health care reimbursement policies allow BMT to become a major profit center for any hospital that successfully establishes a program. Patient care costs of research have traditionally been paid by insurers, so any researchers in this field must advocate for reimbursement of these procedures. Since there is no national and virtually no state policy that supports payment for these costs as research beneficial to society, this advocacy simultaneously facilities nonresearch exploitation of the technology for monetary gain. A "for-profit" company has even been established to exploit this policy failure. This outcome is wrong, and ultimately damages patients, society as a whole, and future clinical research.

A series of failures of public and professional regulation has brought us to this point, and BMT researchers must share the blame for the present damaging situation. We must redefine appropriate policy in this area, for failure to do so will damage future conduct of clinical research and increase the probability that health care reform will be unable to support this important activity. Premature technology dissemination has been universally recognized as a damaging component of the increased cost of health care. What can be done?

1. Require support but limit reimbursement of BMT patient care costs to research studies. These procedures are extremely costly and technology is evolving rapidly. We can no longer afford to encourage technology dissemination just because a treatment is shown to be superior to established therapy. Until cost-effectiveness is maximized and technology is stabilized, BMT programs should be limited to research centers. Virtually every country except the United States already does this. Travel reimbursement for patients and limited family members living in rural areas should be available to those who wish to participate in these programs.

2. Abolish professional fee-for-service reimbursement for research studies. Instead, professional reimbursement should be based upon research productivity and conduct of IRB-approved protocols, and be capped at a level compatible with public policy concerns. No professional reimbursement for BMT should be available outside of research studies performed in research centers.

3. Establish restrictive criteria for BMT centers. Present criteria of professional societies are inadequate both in terms of required expertise and lack of linkage to research. Certification should be performed by organizations with minimal monetary stake in the review outcome such as Cancer Cooperative Groups. Certification should be available to any center with proven expertise, adequate activity level, and ongoing research productivity as demonstrated by peer-reviewed publications. For new centers and programs seeking approval, below-cost reimbursement could be made available during a probationary period.

All parties with a stake in the outcome of clinical research must sacrifice if we are to nurture improved health care results from high technology treatments without severely affecting health care costs. Cancer researchers and institutions must be willing to limit the profitability of high technology research. Insurers must acknowledge their responsibility to contribute to clinical research since they benefit from its outcome. The public must be willing to endure inconvenience and dislocation if they wish to receive high-technology treatments during the research phase. We cannot afford to deliver these programs in every community hospital. Finally, government must reform statutes that damage these efforts. These include IRB regulations that can be construed as making it unethical to limit care in BMT to research studies, antitrust regulations that might defeat the goals outlined above, and the highly damaging ERISA and related statutes that exempt employers and government from reasonable health care regulation. No accountable health plan should be approved without specific language defining its responsibility to support research studies.

BMT researchers, hematologists, and oncologists have a short time to demonstrate that high-technology BMT treatments can be conducted in a manner that is sensitive to the public interest. If we fail to do so, further pursuit of the most important leads in cancer treatment over the past decade will be conducted under policies defined by health plan executives and government bureaucrats. Everyone else will be a loser.

Ms. NORTON. Thank you, Doctor. Dr. Champlin.

Dr. CHAMPLIN. I am here representing myself, as well as the American Society of Blood and Marrow Transplantation, a professional organization representing about 450 physicians and scientists involved in the field of blood and marrow transplantation. It is important to note this field is probably one of the most rapidly-moving in all of medicine.

The effectiveness, the safety, the cost-effectiveness of this procedure have grown dramatically over the last decade where we have seen better results in terms of patient responses and survival, lower risks to the patients, lower risks in terms of mortality, and in the last several years, rapid reductions in the cost of the procedure both with advances in technology and with the pressures of managed care environment.

In my prepared remarks, I have summarized the results of this procedure as have other speakers. I will only briefly summarize them again. But if you look over at the thousands of patients that have now received transplants, either bone marrow or blood stem cells, it is clear given higher doses of chemotherapy in patients sensitive to chemotherapy does increase their response. You cannot be cured of the disease if you do not get a complete response; and you can double the complete response rate by giving this treatment.

Most patients with stage four disease will relapse within a relatively short period of time. There is approximately a 20 percent of the patients surviving beyond five years. That is not expected with any other therapy. I included in my submission 10 patients in our group of about 140 that are going on five years, five to eight years in continuous disease-free status.

Most likely patients to benefit are those that had a good response to standard therapy. In that group we have about 40 percent of the patients who achieved a completed remission with standard treatment still alive and protected survival beyond five to eight years after the high dose treatment.

The third page of my presentation is from Dr. Peters' article where you see the disease-free survival, survival without recurrence of breast cancer patients, the high stage two patients, where his curve plateaus at about 70 percent is clearly at the non-randomized comparative groups selected from these studies where in five years 30 percent of those people were alive and disease-free.

I think it is fair to say this is probably the most promising treatment that has been published in the last decade in the field of breast cancer. Clearly one that the patients are aware of as you heard from the testimony here today. Clearly this is a type of treatment that needs to be further evaluated.

I actually agree with Dr. Henderson that definitive proof is needed in terms of the efficacy of this treatment and these randomized trials are important to do that. It is also clear this is an increasingly promising treatment and patients should have access to this therapy.

I personally believe that they should be able to participate in the phase one/two trials that do not require annualization to an untreated group. If the patients prefer to be treated in this fashion, it is the opinion of their physicians to refer them as such and there are important and critical studies being done looking at innovations both in the administration of therapy and supporting care measures and handling of the blood and bone marrow transplants themselves to further improve these therapies.

Clearly this is a moving field. It is not fair to say marrow transplants is just one treatment. It is one approach to treatment where there is a variety of approaches that could improve it even further. These new approaches do in fact need to be studied.

One of our problems in medicine in general is that the medical insurance industry looks at things as black and white. Either they are experimental or they are standard care. There is nothing in between. If it is experimental, they do not pay for it, it shouldn't be done. If it is standard care, everybody can do it and it is a treatment set in stone.

But clearly bone marrow transplants are something in between. This is a developing therapy, clearly a promising developmental therapy. All of the speakers, including my two colleagues at the moment, have indicated that this is a field where we need to be conducting further clinical research and clinical trials.

Clinical trials, I think the term is even sort of bandied about in a way that is perhaps misleading. Being on a clinical trial means that one is doing something with a prospective plan and collecting data in a way that you can interpret the results. Clearly, no one would argue this is not a laudable goal with any new treatment where we are trying to define where it should be used, who it could be used optimally, what would be its relative role versus alternative treatments.

All the speakers this morning have supported the concept patients getting a new treatment or developing therapy-like bone marrow transplants should be participating in clinical trials so their experience can go on to a greater understanding of the field and being able to move it forward in an even more effective fashion. The reluctance of the insurance industry to cover this procedure has led to much of the political division that we have heard today.

In my State of Texas, the Attorney General of the State of Texas sued a major insurance company for its failure to cover breast cancer. That company capitulated and is now offering this as a covered service. Another State where it has been discussed now requires it by statute for citizens of its State.

Clearly there is a national demand for access to the service based upon promising clinical results. Think about insurance, insurance for your home, your car, or medical insurance. It is there to protect you from catastrophic events like cancer, like your home burning down. This is something that should be there to help you when you need it most where you could not afford the care otherwise.

That is why I personally think it is catastrophic indeed when your insurance carrier at the time that you need them most turns you away saying we will not pay for expensive therapy; we will limit your coverage to cheap treatments. In fact, we have seen insurance carriers developing products where they would preclude patients from receiving any sort of transplant, a kidney transplant, liver transplant or bone marrow transplant as part of the coverage. This is an attractive proposal to a young person, 20-years-old, looking to save money anywhere you can. You do not think you will ever need a transplant operation.

But of course when the time comes, it is then too late to change your insurance to something that would cover it; and very often, the taxpayer is the one who is left to shoulder the burden if the patient is then treated on medicaid or through other funds not subsidized through their own insurance policies.

So I want this committee to give instructions to your own insurance carrier to indeed cover this service; perhaps this and other promising treatments that do require further evaluation, but are clearly a benefit to patients and clearly should be covered in the scheme of health care.

[The prepared statement of Dr. Champlin follows:]

PREPARED STATEMENT OF DR. RICHARD CHAMPLIN, PRESIDENT OF THE AMERICAN SOCIETY FOR BLOOD AND BONE MARROW TRANSPLANTS, HOUSTON

SUMMARY OF CONSIDERATIONS FOR HIGH DOSE CHEMOTHERAPY FOR BREAST CANCER

Breast cancer is a leading cause of mortality in young women. This disease does respond to chemotherapy but is rarely cured once spread beyond the original site and less than half of patients with early local breast cancer with spread to involve more than 10 local lymph glands live without relapse for 5 years.

Several thousand patients have received high dose chemotherapy with autologous bone marrow or blood stem cell transplants. This is now the most frequent indication for high dose chemotherapy. We have documented that the chance of achieving a complete remission is doubled in patients receiving high dose chemotherapy and approximately 20% of patients with metastatic cancer survive disease free >5 years. Over 1000 patients have received high dose therapy for high risk stage 2 disease and >70% are projected to remain disease free beyond 5 years. This is clearly the most important therapy for breast cancer which remains with a grim prognosis with alternative therapies. These results far exceed any other reported treatment for breast cancer patients. Further research and development is needed for this form of treatment and the role of high dose therapy vs. standard dose chemotherapy needs to be further defined in controlled trials. It is clear that this is a highly active therapy which is most likely to produce a complete remission and offers a curative potential for this usually fatal disease.

With increasing experience, the procedure is becoming safer and less expensive. In recent studies treatment related mortality has been reduced to 1–5%, and the cost of the procedure has been reduced to $60,000 to $100,000. This compares favorably for cost effectiveness with other modern therapies.

The available data justifies routine coverage of high dose chemotherapy for appropriately selected patients (age <60, no comorbid diseases, tumor sensitive to standard dose chemotherapy or in remission after surgery). Patients should be treated in centers experienced and skilled in delivering the therapy and should participate in clinical studies to further improve this form of therapy or phase III studies to define its relative role vs. alternative treatments.

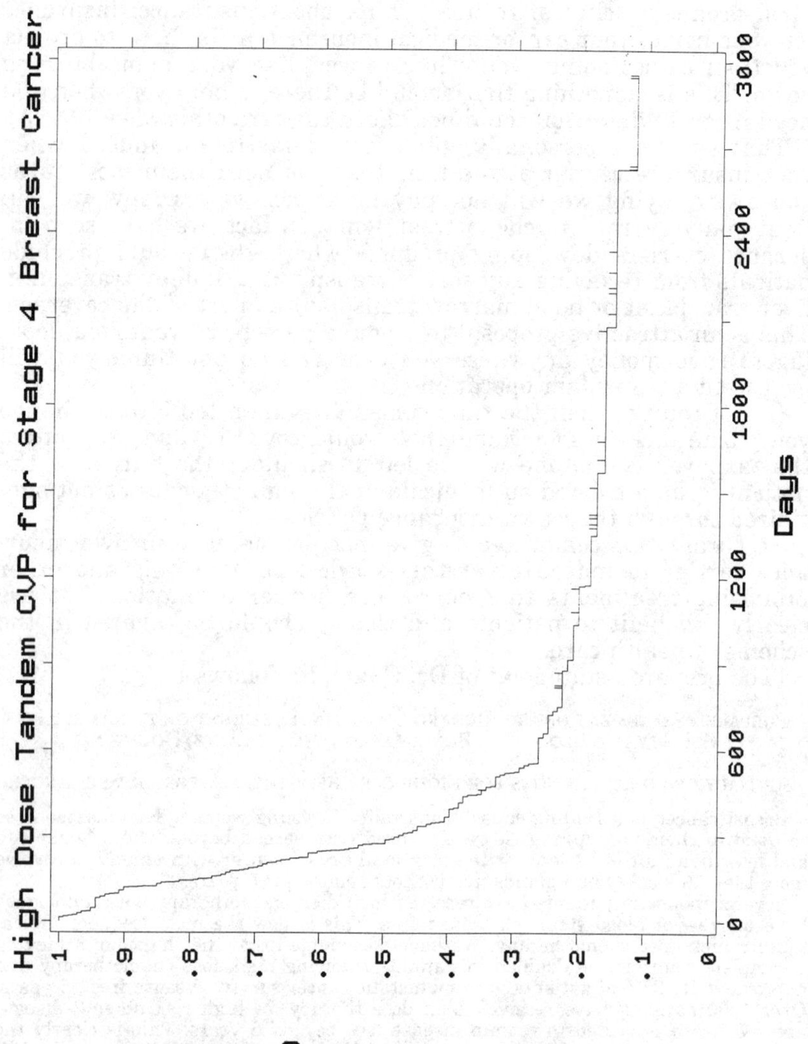

High Dose Tandem CVP for Stage 4 Breast Cancer
Freedom From Progression
Days
1
.9
.8
.7
.6
.5
.4
.3
.2
.1
0
0
600
1200
1800
2400
3000

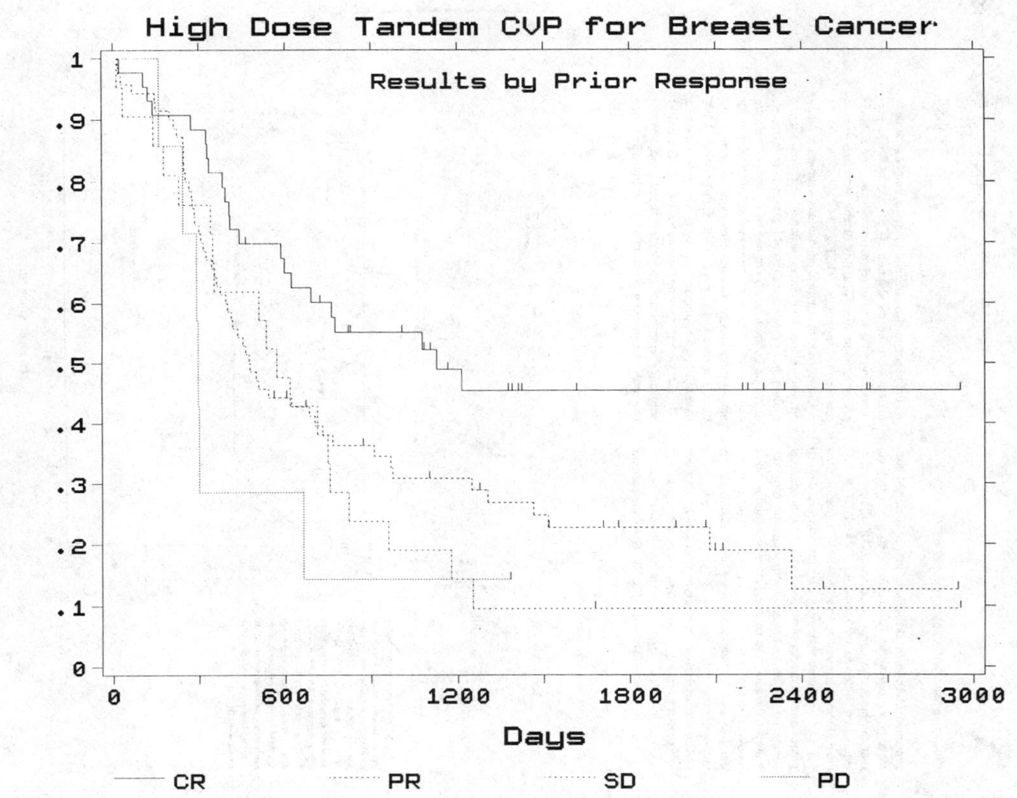

High Dose Tandem CVP for Breast Cancer
Results by Prior Response
Probability of Survival
Days
CR
PR
SD
PD

generated enthusiasm, skepticism, new studies, and controversy. We present here data using a sequential program that combines traditional outpatient CAF adjuvant chemotherapy followed by high-dose CPA/cDDP/BCNU chemotherapy consolidation with ABMS, radiation therapy, and hormonal therapy in patients with well-defined pretreatment characteristics. These data show an apparent benefit for the entire high-dose consolidation program; however, the data must be interpreted with caution, since follow-up duration remains short, the study is not randomized, and the treatment carries substantial morbidity and mortality.

The actuarial event-free survival probability (defined as freedom from any local or systemic relapse or early or late therapy-related death) determined by product-limit estimates is 72% at 30 months (Fig 2B). Given the evolving nature of supportive care, and the reduction of treatment toxicity since the introduction of CSF-primed PBPC, presentation of the time to relapse is relevant. The Kaplan-Meier estimate for probability of any local or systemic relapse at 30 months is 19% (Fig 2A).

Comparison to historical populations is subject to many potential biases. Differences in patient selection, staging evaluation, age, hormone receptor status, dose-intensity, follow-up duration, and unknown factors may complicate comparisons. However, the prognosis of patients with high-risk primary breast cancer involving 10 or more axillary lymph nodes is poor in all reported series.[15] We have selected for comparison patients treated over the past 17 years on previous and concurrent CALGB trials of adjuvant chemotherapy for primary breast cancer. While two trials used different chemotherapy programs and were

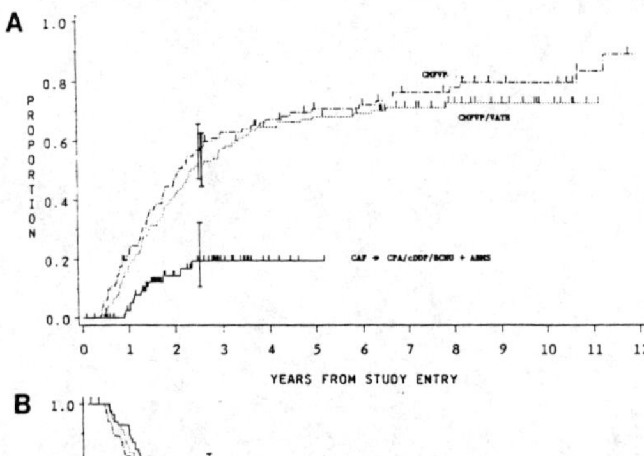

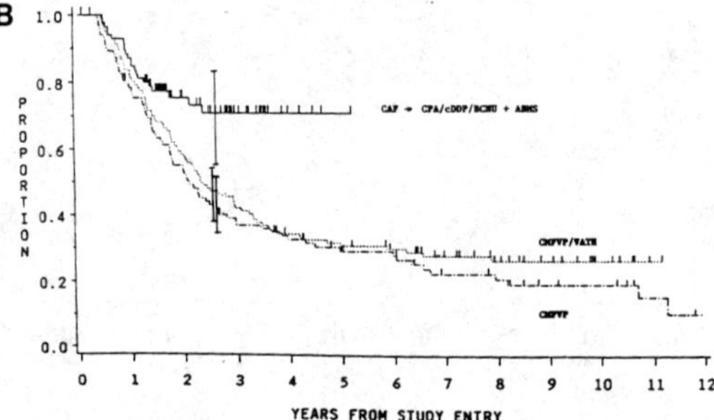

Fig 2. (A) Actuarial probability of relapse or (B) event-free survival for eligible and treated patients (CAF → CPA/cDDP/BCNU + ABMT) and for similar patients selected from two trials using adjuvant CMFVP (CALGB 7581) or CMFVP/VATH (CALGB 8082). Vertical bars represent the 95% confidence intervals for each data set determined at 30 months. Tick marks indicate censored events.

Dose-Intensive Therapy with Autologous Bone Marrow Transplantation for Treatment of Breast Cancer

RICHARD CHAMPLIN, MD

High-dose chemotherapy with hematopoietic support is increasingly used for the treatment of advanced breast cancer. This review summarizes the basic concepts of dose intensity, the principles of autologous bone marrow and blood stem cell transplantation, the clinical results to date, and future directions using this approach in breast cancer.

Concepts of Dose Intensity

Chemotherapeutic agents exhibit a dose-dependent antitumor response: increasing the dose results in increased cytotoxicity. The dose response of antimetabolites plateaus at the point of maximal inhibition of the targeted metabolic pathway, but DNA-damaging agents, such as alkylating agents, continue to have a clear dose-response effect across a broad range of levels.[1,2] Dose-intensive therapy for most active agents is limited by myelosuppression, and for those agents, use of autologous marrow or blood stem cell transplantation supports substantial dose escalation. For tumors with a steep dose-response curve (Figure 1), dose escalation can have a major impact in cytoreduction. This approach is not useful, however, for chemotherapy-insensitive disease, for which little increase in response can be achieved even with marked dose escalation.

Richard Champlin, MD, Section of Bone Marrow Transplantation, The University of Texas M. D. Anderson Cancer Center, Houston, Texas.

DOSE-INTENSIVE chemotherapy with autologous marrow or blood progenitor cell transplantation is increasingly used for treatment of breast cancer. In patients responding to standard-dose chemotherapy, high-dose alkylating agent therapy results in complete remission in >50% of patients and an approximate 20% prolonged disease-free survival. Up to 80% of patients receiving transplants as adjuvant therapy for high-risk local-regional breast cancer have survived 5 years without recurrence in uncontrolled studies; however, controlled trials are necessary to define the optimal role of this approach. Use of hematopoietic growth factors and peripheral blood progenitor cells accelerates recovery, which reduces costs and the risk of fatal complications.

Cancer Bull 1993;45:532–537
©1993 The University of Texas M. D. Anderson Cancer Center

Autologous Marrow and Blood Stem Cell Transplantation

Normal hematopoietic progenitor cells can be collected either from the bone marrow or peripheral blood. These cells transiently circulate and home to the marrow-restoring hematopoiesis, rescuing the patient from severe and prolonged myelosuppression.[3,4]

Bone marrow is harvested by multiple aspirations under general anesthesia, typically collecting 2 to 3 × 10⁸ nucleated bone marrow cells per kilogram. The cells are cryopreserved using programmed freezing in a cryo-protectant, such as dimethylsulfoxide. When maintained in liquid nitrogen, these cells remain viable and capable of reconstituting hematopoiesis when reinfused intravenously <8 years later. Following myeloablative doses of chemotherapy or total-body irradiation, profound pancytopenia occurs. Peripheral neutrophil and platelet counts fall to near zero levels, remaining at a nadir for approximately 2 weeks before recovering from the reinfused bone marrow cells. Typically, granulocytes recover to >0.5 × 10⁹/L at approximately 21 days after reinfusion of the autologous bone marrow. Platelets generally recover to >20 × 10⁹/L by day 28.[5]

Stem cells and progenitors capable of reconstituting hematopoiesis can be collected from the peripheral blood by repeated leukopheresis.[6] Eight to 12 daily leukophereses are required to collect an adequate cell dose (3 to 5 × 10⁸ mononuclear cells per kilogram) for transplantation.[6] Circulating progenitors can be mobilized, however, by collection during the recovery phase following cytoreduction and after growth factor stimulation using granulocyte colony-stimulating factor (G-CSF) or granulocyte-macrophage colony-stimulating factor (GM-CSF).[7-9] Other factors alone or in combination may be more effective for mobilization.[10]

Peripheral blood progenitors offer an alternative source of hematopoietic cells for transplantation and an effective approach for patients who cannot undergo marrow harvest (such as those who have received pelvic irradiation or those patients who have bone marrow or extensive bone in-

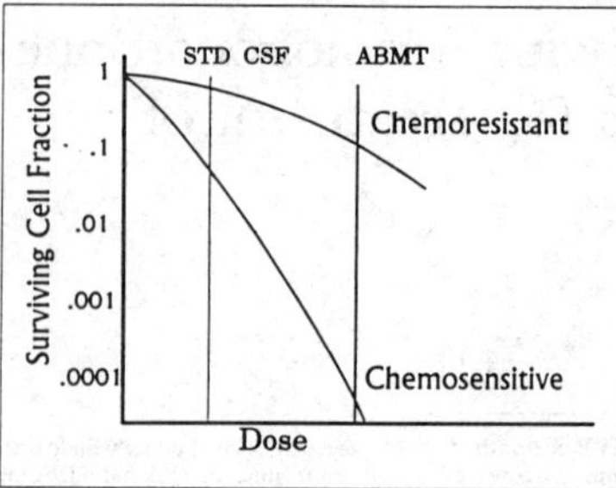

*Figure 1. Dose response to chemotherapy with alkylating agents provides rationale for high-dose regimen. Modest dose escalation can be achieved with colony-stimulating factor (**CSF**) therapy to accelerate neutrophil recovery. Further increase in myelosuppression requires infusion of hematopoietic progenitors from marrow (autologous bone marrow transplantation [**ABMT**]) or peripheral blood to regenerate hematopoiesis. In patients with chemotherapy-sensitive tumors, increasing the dose produces a marked increase in cytoreduction. In patients with chemotherapy-resistant disease, dose escalation has only a modest effect and no clinical benefit. **STD** indicates standard dose.*

volvement, which would likely contaminate a pelvic bone marrow harvest). It remains to be determined if the level of contaminating malignant cells is lower in the peripheral blood compared with the marrow in these patients. Interestingly, autologous transplantation using peripheral blood cells or peripheral blood in addition to marrow has produced somewhat faster hematopoietic recovery of both granulocytes and platelets than autologous marrow transplants in many series.[9]

The major risks of high-dose chemotherapy are nonhematopoietic regimen–related toxicity and severe infection during the granulocytopenic period post-transplant. Severe regimen-related toxicity may occur, particularly in heavily pretreated patients, patients with impaired organ function or poor performance status, and patients with progressive malignancy.[11] Patients with prolonged pancytopenia have increased hepatic and renal abnormalities compared to patients with rapid regeneration of hematopoiesis, consistent with the concept that granulocytes are important in tissue repair.[3] Toxicities vary depending on the chemotherapeutic agents involved, and regimens are designed to include agents with additive cytotoxicity against the malignancy but with nonoverlapping toxicity to allow maximal dose intensity. In early studies, up to 20% of patients typically succumbed to treatment-related mortality. With the development of more

tolerable regimens, improved supportive care including use of hematopoietic growth factors to accelerate granulocyte recovery, and more appropriate patient selection, treatment-related mortality has been reduced to approximately 5% in most series.

Both G-CSF and GM-CSF have been extensively studied to accelerate recovery of hematopoiesis after high-dose chemotherapy alone or with autologous marrow transplantation.[12,13] Granulocyte recovery was significantly accelerated with each factor; there was no change in recovery of platelets or erythrocytes. Following high-dose chemotherapy, neither G-CSF nor GM-CSF affects the depth of the granulocyte nadir or the duration of the period with granulocytes $<0.1 \times 10^9/L$. Once early granulocyte regeneration occurs, recovery to 0.5 and $1.0 \times 10^9/L$ is accelerated,[14] resulting in a reduced need for antibiotic therapy and shorter hospital stays.[15] Delayed platelet recovery remains a major problem, requiring continued platelet transfusion support and predisposing the patient to bleeding complications. Interleukin-3, interleukin-6, and interleukin-11—alone and in combination—are currently under evaluation to potentially enhance platelet recovery.

Dose Intensity in the Treatment of Breast Cancer

Dose intensity increases the response rate of many active agents for treat-

ment of breast cancer.[16,17] Standard-dose chemotherapy produces a 15% to 25% complete response rate and an overall response rate of 50% to 70% in patients with metastatic breast cancer. With combination chemotherapy involving cyclophosphamide, methotrexate, doxorubicin, and fluorouracil, dose intensification increases overall response rates from 15% to 80%.[17] The interval to progression also lengthens with increasing dose intensity, although not as markedly as response rates.

For patients with estrogen receptor-negative (ER−) or hormone-refractory disease, the median response duration is typically 8 to 12 months, and median survival ranges from 12 to 18 months with <10% disease-free at 5 years. Of 1,582 patients with metastatic breast cancer treated at M. D. Anderson Cancer Center, 245 (15.5%) achieved a complete remission with FAC (a combination of fluorouracil, doxorubicin, and cyclophosphamide), but only 13% of the complete-remission patients (2% of all patients) remained in remission at 5 years.[18]

Some active agents for treatment of breast cancer, such as doxorubicin, methotrexate, and the vinca alkaloids, are limited by toxicities other than myelosuppression and are candidates for only limited dose intensification. One moderately myelosuppressive regimen—cisplatin, etoposide, and cyclophosphamide—was originally given with autologous

Table 1. Response to HDCT-ABMT*

Time Point	% CR	% CR + PR	% Early Death
After induction therapy	30	80	—
After HDCT + ABMT	58	80–100	9
After 3 years	26	NA	NA

*High-dose chemotherapy (**HDCT**) and autologous bone marrow transplantation (**ABMT**) in 306 breast cancer patients responding to standard-dose chemotherapy. **CR** indicates complete response; **PR**, partial response; and **NA**, not available. (Adapted from Armitage and Antman.[4])

bone marrow transplantation (BMT), but this regimen can be supported with hematopoietic growth factors without marrow or blood stem cell infusion.[19,20]

Alkylating agents, nitrosoureas, and platinum derivatives have been effective agents in high-dose chemotherapeutic regimens.[20-24] Resistance to these agents is not mediated via P-glycoprotein (mdr-1) and is generally not absolute. Escalation of dose can overcome low-level resistance.[2] Alkylating agents with nonoverlapping toxicities can be combined for additive antitumor effects. Table 1 summarizes clinical results with high-dose chemotherapeutic regimens for metastatic breast cancer.

Minimal Residual Disease

A potential limitation of autologous BMT is the possible involvement of the bone marrow by the malignancy. Breast cancer frequently involves the bone marrow, but standard diagnostic techniques are relatively insensitive in identifying bone marrow metastases. However, more sensitive assays have recently been proposed.

Using monoclonal antibodies directed at cell surface antigens of breast cancer cells and flow cytometry or immunoperoxidase techniques, many patients with newly diagnosed clinically stage I or II breast cancer were shown to have occult bone marrow involvement[25-27]; this finding was associated with a relatively poor prognosis and a short disease-free interval.[27-29] Up to 28% of patients with normal marrow biopsies by light microscopy were positive by immunocytochemical methods. Other studies reported that in 40 to 57% of similar

patients, tumor cells can be grown in tissue culture.[27] Breast cancer cells may also be present in the peripheral blood, and it is unknown whether autologous marrow or peripheral blood transplants would be more likely to be involved by the disease.

Purging and Stem Cell Selection

The clinical implications of occult bone marrow or peripheral blood involvement on the risk of breast cancer relapse following autologous transplantation are unknown, but malignant cells capable of forming marrow metastases may be able to re-establish the malignancy following reinfusion with the autologous hematopoietic cells. Approximately 10^{10} bone marrow cells are collected in a typical harvest; if 0.1% are malignant, 10^7 breast cancer cells would be present in the collection. A number of methods have been proposed to eliminate or "purge" malignant cells, including treatment with antitumor monoclonal antibodies, antibody-toxin conjugates, chemotherapy, or physical techniques.[30-33] These techniques are capable of a 99% to 99.9% (2- to 3-log) reduction of target cells, but this might be insufficient to eliminate all malignant cells. The number and characteristics of breast cancer cells required to produce systemic relapse is unknown.

An alternative method to purging is positively selecting hematopoietic stem cells. CD34-positive cells represent <1% of the bone marrow but encompass progenitors capable of reconstituting hematopoiesis.[34] These cells can be selectively separated from the remaining marrow by reactivity with a biotinylated anti-CD34 monoclonal antibody and adherence to an

avidin column, by immunomagnetic separation, or by panning.[34,35] Each of these methods yields approximately 1% of the starting cell number, but collects >60% of CD34-positive cells. One problem is nonspecific contamination by CD34-negative cells, which constitute approximately 35% to 50% of the final product. This procedure results in an approximately 2-log reduction of malignant cells. Combination of positive selection of CD34-positive cells with negative depletion of malignant cells would be expected to have an additive effect. We are currently assessing the degree of bone marrow involvement in patients with early and advanced breast cancer and evaluating methods for marrow purging using immunomagnetic separation and treatment with an immunotoxin, as well as assessing the effect of positive selection of stem cells, with or without purging, on the elimination of malignant cells from the bone marrow.

High-Dose Chemotherapy with Autologous Transplantation

The most effective regimens have included combinations of alkylating agents and related drugs including cyclophosphamide, melphalan, thiotepa, carmustine, cisplatin, and carboplatin. The doses of these agents can be typically increased threefold over standard doses with autologous blood or marrow transplantations. Studies in patients with metastatic breast cancer have documented that high-dose combination chemotherapy and autologous transplantation results in higher complete response rates than does standard-dose treatment, and approximately 20% of patients have survived >5 years free of recurrent disease.[19-24,36] Results of multiple studies were recently reviewed by Antman (Table 1). Studies at our institution have demonstrated that FAC chemotherapy followed by two courses of high-dose CVP (cyclophosphamide, etoposide, and cisplatin) is relatively well tolerated; more than half of patients with hormone-refractory metastatic breast cancer achieve a complete remission[22]; the actuarial 5-year survival rate is 35%, and 6 of

23 patients who received transplants >5 years ago remain alive and disease-free. Favorable prognostic factors include responsiveness to standard-dose chemotherapy, limited number of disease sites, absence of liver involvement, and good performance status.

Dose-intensive therapy is most effective in patients with a minimal burden of chemotherapy-sensitive tumor cells. Thus, the optimal use of this approach may be as adjuvant therapy in patients with high-risk primary disease. A recent report of high-dose chemotherapy and autologous BMT as adjuvant therapy for stage II or III disease, with 10 or more positive axillary nodes, showed that approximately 80% of these high-risk patients survived free of relapse at >3 years in an uncontrolled trial.[33] Five-year disease-free survival after standard adjuvant therapy ranges from 25% to 57%.

Limitations in Analysis of Results

It is difficult to directly compare the results of dose-intensive chemotherapy trials with standard-dose trials.[36] Patients referred for dose-intensive chemotherapy must be young (generally <60 years of age), have good organ function and performance status, and must be clinically stable to be transferred to the transplant center. Because patients who did not respond to standard-dose chemotherapy have not been shown to benefit from high-dose chemotherapy, this approach is generally limited to patients with a complete or partial response to standard-dose therapy. Thus, patients receiving high-dose chemotherapy are highly selected in order to offer the procedure to those predicted to benefit most from the treatment. This selection bias tends to improve the apparent results of transplantation by eliminating many patients with a relatively poor prognosis. The selection process precludes direct comparison with the relatively unselected patients receiving standard-dose chemotherapy. Controlled clinical studies are necessary for definitive analysis.

Several prospective randomized studies are ongoing for patients with high-risk local-regional disease to determine if high-dose chemotherapy is beneficial as part of adjuvant treatment. For patients with metastatic disease, high-dose chemotherapy results in a high complete response rate, but the median time to progression remains approximately 1 year. In this situation, neither standard-dose nor high-dose chemotherapy is satisfactory; the highest priority at this time should be to substantially improve the complete response rate and duration of response, rather than to perform controlled trials.

Cost and Reimbursement Considerations

Experimental therapy is a treatment for which the risks and benefits are unknown, and an established treatment is one for which sufficient experience clearly defines the anticipated results. Established systemic therapies for breast cancer are known to have only limited effectiveness, and the need to develop improved therapies is paramount.

Many insurance carriers exclude coverage for experimental therapy and have denied payment for high-dose chemotherapy for breast cancer on this basis, which is inappropriate. More than 1,000 patients with breast cancer have been treated with high-dose chemotherapy, and the risks and benefits are well documented. In nearly every study, the response rate is improved over standard-dose alternatives, and a fraction of patients have achieved prolonged disease-free survival. This treatment is still in the developmental phase and its role vs other treatment options must be established. The use of autologous bone marrow and blood stem cell transplantation for this disease should be restricted to cancer research centers, and all patients should be entered in clinical trials to answer these critical questions.

The cost of high-dose chemotherapy and autologous BMT or peripheral blood stem cell transplantation (generally $100,000 to $150,000) is related primarily to the length of hospitalization for supportive care, blood product transfusions, and antibiotic treatment for infection during granulocytopenia. The typical length of hospitalization was 4 to 5 weeks, recently shortened by approximately 1 week with the use of hematopoietic growth factors.

Recent efforts have centered on transferring a major portion of care to the outpatient clinic. Well-organized outpatient infusion centers can administer dose-intensive treatment to stable patients, and, with rapid hematologic recovery induced by growth factors and peripheral blood stem cells, hospitalization may be necessary only for treatment of neutropenic infection or for major complications. In one preliminary study, costs were reduced by 50% for patients receiving outpatient transplantation. Costs are likely to continue to fall with further technologic advances. If survival benefit or higher cure rates can be documented in controlled trials, the costs mentioned would be in keeping with other accepted high-technology procedures.[37]

Future Directions

Dose intensity is important to achieve the maximal cytoreduction with available chemotherapeutic agents. Strategies to overcome drug resistance mechanisms—such as administration of inhibitors to P-glycoprotein, the product of the multidrug resistance gene—may improve the results of high-dose chemotherapy. The administration of chemoprotectant agents that modify extramedullary toxicity without compromising antitumor effects may improve the therapeutic index of these regimens. Novel classes of drugs, including anthrapyrazoles, topoisomerase I inhibitors, and taxanes, have recently shown efficacy against breast cancer and may be important components of future high-dose combination chemotherapy regimens. Monoclonal antibody–radionuclide immunoconjugates are being evaluated as a means of targeting radiotherapy to the tumor and minimizing systemic toxicity. The dose-limiting toxicity of these agents is typically marrow suppression, and their use may be supported by autologous BMT or blood cell transplantation.

A major limitation with autologous BMT is reliance on a single course of high-dose therapy to eradicate the disease.[38] Kinetic resistance and presence of poorly vascularized tumor masses limit the effectiveness of a single course of therapy but might be overcome by administration of multiple courses. Greater overall dose intensity may be achieved by repeated courses of therapy. The ability to collect large numbers of marrow and peripheral blood hematopoietic cells allows administration of two to four courses of treatment.[39]

The collection of bone marrow or peripheral blood hematopoietic cells offers the potential for ex vivo genetic therapy to improve treatment results. Retroviral marking of the autologous marrow is being studied to demonstrate reconstitution of hematopoiesis by the transplanted bone marrow, as well as to determine the origin of relapse after autologous transplantation.[40] If the retroviral marker is present in the breast cancer, it indicates that malignant cells reinfused in the autologous marrow contributed to the relapse. Transfection of genes for drug resistance, such as *mdr*-1, into normal marrow cells may allow better tolerance to subsequent chemotherapy with agents such as doxorubicin, vinca alkaloids, and paclitaxel (Taxol).[41] Alternative strategies include transfection of cytokine genes into hematopoietic cells for enhanced delivery to the tumor, or ex vivo activation of bone marrow or blood lymphoid effector cells to eliminate minimal residual disease.

Finally, dose-intensive therapies must be integrated with other modalities into the overall treatment of breast cancer. This treatment is most likely to be curative if administered at a time of minimal tumor burden and before evolution of drug resistance. The ideal timing should be as adjuvant therapy in high-risk patients with local-regional disease and in patients with complete responses to standard-dose chemotherapy for metastatic disease. Relapse remains a major problem, and use of biologic or immunologic therapies for minimal residual breast cancer after autologous transplantation needs to be evaluated.

References

1. Frei E III, Antman K, Teicher B, et al. Bone marrow autotransplantation for solid tumors—prospects. *J Clin Oncol.* 1989;7:515–526.
2. Frei E III. Alkylating agent resistance in in vitro studies with human cell lines. *Proc Natl Acad Sci USA.* 1985;82:2158–2162.
3. Deisseroth A, Abrams RA. The role of autologous stem cell reconstitution in intensive therapy for resistant neoplasms. *Cancer Treat Rep.* 1979;63:461–471.
4. Armitage JO, Antman KH. *High Dose Cancer Therapy: Pharmacology, Hematopoietins, Stem Cells.* Baltimore, Md: Williams & Wilkins; 1992.
5. Champlin RE, Gale RP. Role of bone marrow transplantation in the treatment of hematologic malignancies and solid tumors: critical review of syngeneic, autologous and allogeneic transplants. *Cancer Treat Rep.* 1984;68:145–161.
6. Kessinger A, Armitage JO. The evolving role of autologous peripheral stem cell transplantation following high-dose therapy for malignancies. *Blood.* 1991;77:211–213. Editorial.
7. Socinski MA, Elias A, Schnipper L, et al. Granulocyte-macrophage colony stimulating factor expands the circulating haemopoietic progenitor cell compartment in man. *Lancet.* 1988;1:1194–1197.
8. Siena S, Bregni M, Brando B, et al. Circulation of CD34⁺ hematopoietic stem cells in the peripheral blood of high-dose cyclophosphamide-treated patients: enhancement by intravenous recombinant human granulocyte-macrophage colony-stimulating factor. *Blood.* 1989;74:1905–1914.
9. Sheridan WP, Begley CG, Juttner CA, et al. Effect of peripheral-blood progenitor cells mobilised by filgrastim (G-CSF) on platelet recovery after high-dose chemotherapy. *Lancet.* 1992;339:640–644.
10. Geissler K, Valent P, Mayer P, et al. Recombinant human interleukin-3 expands the pool of circulating hematopoietic progenitor cells in primates—synergism with recombinant human granulocyte/macrophage colony-stimulating factor. *Blood.* 1990;75:2305–2310.
11. Bearman SI, Appelbaum FR, Buckner CD, et al. Regimen-related toxicity in patients undergoing bone marrow transplantation. *J Clin Oncol.* 1988;6:1562–1568.
12. Sheridan WP, Morstyn G, Wolf M, et al. Granulocyte colony-stimulating factor and neutrophil recovery after high-dose chemotherapy and autologous bone marrow transplantation. *Lancet.* 1989;2:891–895.
13. Peters WP. Use of cytokines during prolonged neutropenia associated with autologous bone marrow transplantation. *Rev Infect Dis.* 1991;13:993–996.
14. Taylor KM, Jagannath S, Spitzer G, et al. Recombinant human granulocyte colony-stimulating factor hastens granulocyte recovery after high-dose chemotherapy and autologous bone marrow transplantation in Hodgkin's disease. *J Clin Oncol.* 1989;7:1791–1799.
15. Nemunaitis J, Rabinowe SN, Singer JW, et al. Recombinant granulocyte-macrophage colony-stimulating factor after autologous bone marrow transplantation for lymphoid cancer. *N Engl J Med.* 1991;324:1773–1778.
16. Hortobagyi GN, Dunphy F, Buzdar AU, Spitzer G. Dose intensity studies in breast cancer—autologous bone marrow transplantation. *Prog Clin Biol Res.* 1990;354B:195–209.
17. Hryniuk WM. Integrating the concept of dose intensity into a strategy for systemic therapy of malignant disease. *Prog Clin Biol Res.* 1990;354B:93–101.
18. Hortobagyi GN, Frye D, Buzdar AU, et al. Complete remissions in metastatic breast cancer: a thirteen year follow-up report. *Proc Am Soc Clin Oncol.* 1988;7:37. Abstract.
19. Huan SD, Yau JC, Dunphy FR, et al. Impact of autologous bone marrow infusion on hematopoietic recovery after high-dose cyclophosphamide, etoposide, and cisplatin. *J Clin Oncol.* 1991;9:1609–1617.
20. Neidhart JA. Dose-intensive treatment of breast cancer supported by granulocyte-macrophage colony-stimulating factor (GM-CSF). *Breast Cancer Res Treat.* 1991;20(suppl):S15–S23.
21. Peters WP. Dose intensification using combination alkylating agents and autologous bone marrow support in the treatment of primary and metastatic breast cancer: a review of the Duke Bone Marrow Transplantation Program experience. *Prog Clin Biol Res.* 1990;354B:185–194.
22. Dunphy FR, Spitzer G, Buzdar AU, et al. Treatment of estrogen receptor negative or hormonally refractory breast

cancer with double high-dose chemotherapy intensification and bone marrow support. *J Clin Oncol.* 1990;8:1207–1216.

23. Williams SF, Mick R, Desser R, et al. High-dose consolidation therapy with autologous stem cell rescue in stage IV breast cancer. *J Clin Oncol.* 1989;7: 1824–1830.

24. Antman K, Gale R. Advanced breast cancer: high-dose chemotherapy and bone marrow autotransplants. *Ann Intern Med.* 1988;108:570–574.

25. Redding WH, Monaghean P, Imrie SF, et al. Detection of micrometastasis in patients with primary breast cancer. *Lancet.* 1983;2:1271–1274.

26. Giai M, Natoli C, Sismondi P, et al. Bone marrow micrometastases detected by a monoclonal antibody in patients with breast cancer. *Anticancer Res.* 1990;10:119–122.

27. Mann SL, Joshi SS, Weisenburger DD, et al. Detection of tumor cells in histologically normal marrow of autologous transplant patients using culture techniques. *Exp Hematol.* 1986;14:541. Abstract.

28. Mansi JL, Berger U, McDonnell T, et al. The fate of bone marrow micrometastases in patients with primary breast cancer. *J Clin Oncol.* 1989;7:445–449.

29. Cote RJ, Rosen PP, Lesser ML, et al. Prediction of early relapse in patients with operable breast cancer by detection of occult bone marrow micrometastases. *J Clin Oncol.* 1991;9:1749–1756.

30. Bjorn MJ, Manger R, Sivam G, et al. Selective elimination of breast cancer cells from human bone marrow using an antibody–*Pseudomonas* exotoxin A conjugate. *Cancer Res.* 1990;50:5992–5996.

31. Shpall EJ, Bast RC, Joines WT, et al. Immunomagnetic purging of breast cancer from bone marrow for autologous transplantation. *Bone Marrow Transplant.* 1991;7:145–151.

32. Vredenburgh JJ, Simpson W, Memoli VA, Ball ED. Reactivity of anti-CD15 monoclonal antibody PM-81 with breast cancer and elimination of breast cancer cells from human bone marrow by PM-81 and immunomagnetic beads. *Cancer Res.* 1991;51:2451–2455.

33. O'Briant KC, Shpall EJ, Houston LL, et al. Elimination of clonogenic breast cancer cells from human bone marrow: a comparison of immunotoxin treatment with chemoimmunoseparation using 4-hydroperoxycyclophosphamide, monoclonal antibodies, and magnetic microspheres. *Cancer.* 1991;68:1272–1278.

34. Civin CI, Strauss LC, Fackler MJ, et al. Positive stem cell selection: basic science. *Prog Clin Biol Res.* 1990;333:387–402.

35. Berenson RJ, Bensinger WI, Hill RS, et al. Engraftment after infusion of CD34⁺ marrow cells in patients with breast cancer or neuroblastoma. *Blood.* 1991;77: 1717–1722.

36. Eddy DM. High-dose chemotherapy with autologous bone marrow transplantation for the treatment of metastatic breast cancer. *J Clin Oncol.* 1992;10: 657–670.

37. Hillner BE, Smith TJ, Desch CE. Efficacy and cost-effectiveness of autologous bone marrow transplantation in metastatic breast cancer: estimates using decision analysis while awaiting clinical trial results. *JAMA.* 1992;267:2055–2061.

38. Korn EL, Simon R. Selecting dose-intense drug combinations: metastatic breast cancer. *Breast Cancer Res Treat.* 1992;20:155–166.

39. Tepler I, Cannistra SA, Frei E, et al. Use of peripheral blood progenitor cells abrogates the myelotoxicity of repetitive outpatient high-dose carboplatin and cyclophosphamide chemotherapy. *J Clin Oncol.* 1993;11:1583–1591.

40. Brenner MK, Rill DR, Moen RC, et al. Gene-marking to trace origin of relapse after autologous bone-marrow transplantation. *Lancet.* 1993;341:85–86.

41. Sorrentino BP, Brandt SJ, Bodine D, et al. Selection of drug-resistant bone marrow cells in vivo after retroviral transfer of human *MDR1. Science.* 1992;257: 99–103.

Ms. NORTON. Thank you very much, Dr. Champlin.

Let me begin by asking Dr. Henderson, given the state of the data now, would it be an inappropriate thing for patients on an individualized basis to be treated with HDC/ABMT treatment by NCI-approved institutions like Sloan or Georgetown, you name one?

Dr. HENDERSON. I believe it would be inappropriate.

Ms. NORTON. Could you explain why? Of course, you know that—you heard testimony perhaps earlier that Sloan, in fact, is administering such treatment.

Dr. HENDERSON. Yes, but that doesn't make it right. Sloan–Kettering was one of the leaders in advocating the radical mastectomy a long time after a lot of the country abandoned that approach. No single physician, no single institution, no matter how widely or highly regarded they are perceived, has a monopoly on truth or the right answers. Doctors, doctors collectively have many times and we as a society have many times made very serious errors that have been costly. This is one which I believe there is not evidence that the therapy is even as good as the standard treatment and I think it must be fully evaluated.

There are many institutions including Duke, including the Dana-Farber Cancer Institute, the University of California San Francisco where I am now that will not permit patients to be treated with high dose chemotherapy and bone marrow transplant unless they are on a formal study.

At the heart of that formal study is an informed consent. That informed consent should say this is an investigational treatment and should indicate what is known and what is not known as a— as objectively as possible. I find it very interesting that when—that the public debate on tomoxafin recently placed great emphasis on informed consent while here I don't think people are too concerned about that.

Ms. NORTON. What gives you that impression?

Dr. HENDERSON. Everything I see in the newspapers, the various public arguments that have taken place over the last several months as we have been debating the tamoxifen issues. It seems we are on——

Ms. NORTON. That is what I am asking. What have you heard that anywhere indicates that the women who would, in fact, be treated would not be aware that, and be asked to give their informed consent about, a treatment that is new? What gives you that impression?

Dr. HENDERSON. Five of the women who testified this morning. I felt in each case—and I think this is natural and perfectly acceptable—but at this point their perception in my view is not consistent with the evidence that exists. In other words, their perception is they are alive because of bone marrow transplant. We do not have such evidence. They very likely or very plausibly would be alive without it. There is no one who can look into a crystal ball and say you will be dead in two years without this therapy, with it, you will be alive. That is not possible.

Ms. NORTON. You do concede that there is some data showing the efficacy of this treatment among some women?

Dr. HENDERSON. No. I would not say there is evidence this has greater or equal efficacy among any group of women.

Ms. NORTON. OPM has asserted there is no medical consensus. From the testimony from the three of you, I detect that that may well be the case. I would like the other two witnesses to comment on your last statement.

Dr. CHAMPLIN. I am a person who has treated breast cancer both with standard chemotherapy and bone marrow transplants. My interest is in the marrow transplant field. I take a different view than Dr. Henderson. I think if you look at the curve in the figure that I provided to you in my written statement, that clearly this is a treatment where the preliminary data at least in the stage two patients is extremely promising. I personally cannot conceive of any patient selection or other factors that could have resulted in that appearing to be better than the control group to such an extent other than the fact that this is an effective treatment.

Also, I agree we need further treatment to clarify its role versus alternative therapies. We and others are working to make the treatment less toxic, safer and less expensive. There have been tremendous advances in that regard where the mortality of the procedure now is in fact routinely less than 5 percent and more in the 1 percent range for the patients in excellent physical condition. The treatment is certainly safer than it has been. At least the results as we can see them up to five years looks extremely promising. Where the slope of the relapse curve is reduced in a way that would suggest there is a marked improvement in the natural history and probably an improvement in the cure factor. You will need 20 years to know about curing breast cancer. During that time, a lot of patients are at risk to die from this disease. So the question in what we as physicians always have to sum up and contend with is on the basis of the information that is available to us today, what would we recommend to a patient.

I personally am quite comfortable in recommending they participate in clinical trials involving bone marrow transplantation, both randomized trials as well as the phase one and two studies to try to improve upon this promising treatment. I personally think it is very important that the health care system support a woman's access to this and other types of promising treatments.

Ms. NORTON. Dr. Jones.

Dr. JONES. I would like to associate myself substantially with Dr. Champlin's remarks. I would make a few points to draw points of consensus between us rather than differences. I think all of us are saying that we think this is a promising treatment but perhaps the critical element is the involvement of patients.

Ms. NORTON. Dr. Henderson does not say it is promising. He says it may be worse than conventional treatment.

Dr. JONES. I think even Dr. Henderson would say there is promise to it, but would take the point of argument as to whether there is concrete evidence it is superior. Dr. Champlin and I may feel the weight of the evidence suggests it is superior. We all agree the randomized or coin-flip trials are essential for definitive proof. Perhaps where I take some other exception is that I just think that with the wide range of peer reviewed NCI-funded trials that are available, that the patient care costs for trials outside of the coin-flip trials should also be made available by insurers, else why should the NCI be funding these other activities if they didn't think they were meritorious. One essential element of these trials is they will only be approved by the institutional review boards at the institutions on the context that there is evidence to suggest that there is no superior treatment.

It is important to draw the distinction between proof it is superior. It just says we are doing these studies, there has to be a reason to believe there is no superior treatment to what is available at the time. So the full range of these studies seem to me to be meritorious.

Ms. NORTON. Where would you say is the weight of opinion here? Dr. Henderson's opinion seems to be fairly conservative. Yours seems to be less so. I am looking now for the weight of opinion of the scientific community.

Dr. HENDERSON. The question you specifically asked me was is there sufficient evidence to treat any group of patients outside of clinical trials. My answer to that question was no.

Ms. NORTON. I am sorry. I didn't hear that.

Dr. HENDERSON. I said the question you asked me, I hope I interpreted it correctly, is is there sufficient evidence to treat patients who wanted outside of clinical trials. My answer to that question was no. I don't believe either of my colleagues have disagreed with that position. We have all stated that there is a consensus——

Ms. NORTON. Just a moment.

Dr. CHAMPLIN. Perhaps I don't precisely agree with that. I personally believe patients should participate in clinical trials when they are developing therapy to try to improve that treatment and collect information necessary to evaluate that therapy. Now there are some patients who have special circumstances in a way that they could not be eligible for a clinical trial because—a clinical trial is set up for the trial. With the idea of defining a group of homogeneous patients from which you can interpret the results, there may be the occasional patient that is a good candidate for a bone marrow transplant that might not meet those eligibility criteria. Under those circumstances they might still be treated with that modality, although the vast majority of patients are in good enough condition that they should, in fact, be eligible for clinical research studies.

So my view is that it is a treatment option that I believe is an appropriate treatment option for a patient but they, within this developing area of therapy, they should be participating in clinical research studies if that is possible.

Ms. NORTON. Dr. Jones?

Dr. JONES. I believe with the broad range of clinical trials that are available at our institutions and others, there are very few patients who are medically appropriate for these treatments for whom a protocol at one institution or the other cannot be found. My personal practice at the University of Colorado is to only treat patients eligible for trials, but that includes trials that do not include the coin-flip provision.

Ms. NORTON. That is really the critical difference, Dr. Henderson. That is what I heard all along.

Dr. HENDERSON. I do not disagree with that. I am not opposed to paying for patients on phase one and phase two trials. I did make the caveat not all trials are equal. There is an awful lot of research going on in this country. It does not apply to what Dr. Jones is doing, but it does in institutions including universities where small numbers of patients are being treated in a way that no question will ever be answered. It is unrealistic for research and is wasting lots of money. In this case, not wasting lots of research money but health care dollars.

You know, I think in general principle we are in agreement. I think even Dr. Jones might agree with that last statement, too. I don't know. The differences are treating patients off those studies and outside of proper trials.

Ms. NORTON. I am going to turn to Mrs. Morella. I don't vote on conference reports. She has to go.

Mrs. MORELLA. See, she is lucky in many ways. Doesn't have to vote on the Journal of the day before; a conference report that we feel will have a lopsided vote.

I am interested in how many research centers are there, Dr. Jones, that you would say would be approved?

Dr. JONES. Probably Dr. Cheson would be a better person to ask that question to. Certainly there are centers within every State or at least within an adjacent State, very small populous States, that fall into the rubric we have been discussing. I think it is clear they are accessible for any patient who wants to go to them for inclusion in these studies.

Mrs. MORELLA. So if you have a research center that has experts and peer review, you would feel as you stated that there should be payment for this treatment?

Dr. JONES. Yes, I do. Maybe I could expand a little bit to illuminate where the concern of all of us is. There is actually existing now a for-profit company whose job is to build bone marrow transplant units—I don't mean to cast too many aspersions—but at Podunk hospitals around the country, to use a phrase used earlier. I think all of us have grave reservations about this.

You have to know a quirk of our insurance system is such that bone marrow transplants for hospitals are profitable. Therefore hospitals will set them up sometimes with inadequate support facilities so they can sometimes make money. All of us are concerned that patients get good quality care. One mark of good quality care are these research studies we have all alluded to.

Dr. HENDERSON. May I add a footnote to that?

Going along with exactly the same point that Dr. Jones just made, when some insurance companies that have decided to pay for patients only on trials have gone to institutions, including versus prestigious institutions, and said we will pay for the patients on your trials, but only under the condition that we pay only the costs. In other words, this isn't like any other hospital bill. This really has to be cut to the bare bones, but we will pay for the hospital costs. You pay for anything that is truly experimental, overhead, so on and all. We will pay for the costs.

There are a number of institutions, based on my own personal experience, that have refused to even discuss that option, to even negotiate. I think it isn't—it is important to recognize that there are lots of motivations in this issue that are very complicated. Repeatedly this morning we have heard that the insurers would do anything just to cut costs or save a dollar. Well, I work with a lot of insurers. They have in almost every case a medical officer who is a physician; and I find those physicians vary from those who have the same driving concern about patients that physicians who practice do, to those who I think are very callous.

Likewise, when I go into the community or work with my fellow—my colleagues, there is a great range among physicians in terms of what is driving them. There are many cases where there are lots of rewards for us as physicians even if they are not monetary. We do have a vestment in this. We have talked about the patient having a vestment. That vestment is in hope. It is a very important vestment. The medical institutions and administrators who run these also have a vested interest. This is not one thing where any single group has the pure motivations and all other groups, you know, have conflicted motivations.

Mrs. MORELLA. I noticed with your testimony, Dr. Henderson, there is testimony from Blue Cross-Blue Shield. Is this because you represent Blue Cross-Blue Shield?

Dr. HENDERSON. I do not represent Blue Cross-Blue Shield. These statements I made are completely my own. I have worked with Blue Cross-Blue Shield but I have worked with Medi-Cal of California, Healthnet, Kaiser, a number of different organizations. As I indicated, all without compensation because I believe strongly there must be physicians willing to try to stand in the midst of this and deal with all the forces rather than taking sides. I tried very carefully not to be polarized.

Mrs. MORELLA. There is a statement by Blue Cross-Blue Shield Association attached. You used the term "capricious", "arbitrary", et cetera. I do not see that there is equity. Why does Blue Cross-Blue Shield pay for it in one area and not pay for it in another area? Why is there this ambiguity, even going beyond the Federal employee health benefit plan?

Dr. CHAMPLIN. Blue Cross-Blue Shield is not one company. They are a federation of independent units. One of their units——

Mrs. MORELLA. They hide behind this idea that if it is experimental, investigatory, all that kind of stuff; yet, there just isn't any agreement?

Dr. CHAMPLIN. I question this thought of experimental. If you think of what is an experiment, experimental treatment is you give a treatment and you do not know what is going to happen. That is an experiment. So when you introduce a new drug that has never been given to a human being before, that is an experiment, clearly an experimental treatment.

We are now in a situation where there have been thousands of patients treated with high dose therapy for breast cancer. There are more than a thousand in the last year. Probably around maybe 5,000 total patients treated, there is no single registry of these individuals. The number is increasing rapidly.

I think not just because of economic questions but because of virtually every major treatment center sees this as a promising direction and offers a program for that treatment to be administered. Clearly it has become a standard of care, if you will, at least in the academic centers, or the tertiary care centers involved in this level of research.

Over the last decade, the insurance industry has come around to cover this in a much greater fashion. Perhaps five years ago, it was an unusual company that would cover it. I think that now 80 percent of insurance companies do cover this. Again, as the data became stronger, that would support the efficacy of this treatment. I see OPM is again behind the pace of the rest of the country and at this point, the majority of insurance carriers will in fact pay for this treatment.

Mrs. MORELLA. I notice you called it the most promising treatment that we have. I was disturbed at a comment that you made, Dr. Henderson, where you said those people who have lived for years after the treatment may well have lived that long without the treatment. I was thinking of not only that treatment but my husband, for instance, had bypass surgery. Would he have lived that long—he continues to live—if he had not had it? I just didn't quite understand that.

Dr. HENDERSON. There is a real question. For example, we spend about $10 billion per year in our society on CABGs, coronary artery bypass graft. There is absolutely no question that for that particular treatment we improve quality of life and survival of selected groups of patients.

But we are spending probably much, much more than we would need to spend, if we had performed proper randomized trials on CABGs back in the sixties rather than letting them become so totally immersed and now it is a very difficult problem. It is always difficult to withdraw therapy once it becomes established. I gave you the example of radical mastectomies. There are hundreds of others in the history of medicine including recent history of medicine.

Mrs. MORELLA. What about the example I gave of the testicular cancer?

Dr. HENDERSON. I was on a panel for approval of that. Okay? I did vote in fact for the approval. I want to emphasize in my remarks that that is a very, very limited indication that patients who are at end stage disease. First of all, testicular cancer is a much, much more responsive tumor to chemotherapy than is breast cancer. Just as leukemia is a much more responsive tumor to chemotherapy than breast cancer.

In the case of testicular cancer, there is no question at this point but what patients with testicular cancer are cured with the use of chemotherapy including conventional dose chemotherapy. The indications of improvement is if a patient has failed three levels of chemotherapy and relapsed each time or a patient has actually had growth of their testicular cancer while receiving chemotherapy, then they are eligible for bone marrow transplant.

I would be willing to bet if we had similar data for breast cancer, and we could define a niche of that type, it would be approved tomorrow by everybody unanimously. We do not have such data.

Mrs. MORELLA. I have to go vote. Thank you very much.

Ms. NORTON. Mr. Myers?

Mr. MYERS. Thank you, Madam Chairwoman. I apologize for missing part of your testimony. There are many responsibilities in the House including voting. I need a cardiologist instead of an oncologist.

Dr. CHAMPLIN. You are in the wrong room.

Mr. MYERS. Not right now anyway.

If BMT is going to be clinically approved, through the clinical trials, would that be the standard primary care in the future?

Dr. CHAMPLIN. My personal view would be that it will be once the clinical trials resolve precisely what categories of patients will benefit, it will be appropriate to be used in that fashion, but not the majority of patients with breast cancer that will be indicated. Most patients, again as Dr. Cheson mentioned, if they have small tumors do not have extensive lymph node involvement, are not presently considered candidates for bone marrow transplantation. Among people with metastatic disease, it is only those that have the most standardized disease that seem to benefit from the high dose treatments. It is likely to be only a fraction of the patients. I think my own personal feeling is that a fraction of the patients are very likely to benefit from this treatment and it should be offered to them.

Mr. MYERS. Any other comments?

Dr. HENDERSON. I personally would bet that in 30 to 40 years— there is going to be a long transition there—but 30 to 40 years from now, I suspect very few breast cancer patients will be getting chemotherapy either low or high dose in the way we know it now. I do not think that my major thrust is to study the disease itself and increasingly I am convinced that the hope of the future is going to be in patients that we are now beginning that are in phase one and that they are going to eventually prove to be much more effective than the cytotoxic or poisons we used in the past generations.

That doesn't mean I don't use those, or don't treat patients with them. That doesn't mean I don't believe it hasn't been a great advance or that these trials should be done. If I am going to bet on the long-term future, that is where I would bet on it. I believe it is as likely as not that few women with breast cancer will be getting a bone marrow transplant 10 years from now if we can complete the studies.

Mr. MYERS. I hope 10, 20 or 30 years we will not have to worry about it. We will know what causes it. I don't know whether it will be environmental or any—I don't know—no one knows that at this point which is prevalent. I hope we find out what causes it and don't worry about it. Like we don't have to worry about many diseases today we worried about 40 years ago.

Dr. JONES. I would add to that by saying I agree with you. We all hope we will have fundamentally less toxic and more effective gene therapy 30 years from now.

I would point out under the present policies OPM and the insurers operated on, we will never get to that point unless we reimburse, because the bottom line is they will not pay for the patient care costs or the trials necessary to get there knowingly based upon the policies they articulate.

I would make a plea to you: It is a vacuum of policy that needs to be addressed. If their standard is we will not pay for any kind of patient care until we are definitively sure it is superior standard treatment, you will not have new care to evaluate because it will never get to that point. Patient care costs for research need to be paid attention to. I plead with you to consider this issue.

Mr. MYERS. Maybe OPM deserves consideration and blame here. How many insurance companies do pay today for ABMT?

Dr. JONES. I agree with Dr. Champlin, most commercial indemnity insurers pay for this.

Blue Cross-Blue Shield of many States, Aetna, Prudential, Metropolitan Life, Mutual of Omaha so on and so forth. In my experience as a predictor of whether an insurer will pay is the type of insurer that they are; that is most commercial indemnity insurers pay. Many, if not the majority, of health maintenance organizations do not pay.

Mr. MYERS. Anyone else?

Dr. HENDERSON. I wanted to comment on that. I know at least Chairwoman Norton is a lawyer. I don't know how many of the rest of you are.

Mr. MYERS. I don't brag about it.

Dr. HENDERSON. My experience with lawyers, one question that lawyers often times raise in a case, is if you are going to take it to trial, what are the possible outcomes? How much will it cost you to get the best outcome? Is that worth it?

I think that we have to recognize that a lot of the insurance companies have gone through this process and decided, first of all, that it is not worth taking to court because they are most likely to lose; and that it is going to be very costly. And secondly, they are very, very sensitive to the PR losses that they face.

There is also competition which, I think, is what we want in our society actually. I am not opposed to that. There is competition among insurers saying well, you know, I am going to offer this in my plan. I don't know that that is particularly bad.

But I just want to emphasize I don't believe the reason why insurers have approved this in many cases is because they are convinced the data are there, or the medical panels are convinced of that, but rather for other reasons that may be totally unrelated to that, including saving money, paying for it rather than fighting it.

Dr. CHAMPLIN. I think to take the other perspective, some of the hesitancy is in fact that this is a common disease, that if you look at the results of bone marrow transplants for uncommon diseases, neuroblastoma in children, for example, is routinely covered by all insurance companies but not as good, and not as promising as breast cancer. If breast cancer was a rare disease, I don't think we would be having this discussion. It is a common disease and affects millions of women. And that it does offer, I believe, the promise to improve the chances of a woman in proper situations of being cured of their disease.

I think it is something that certainly should be available as a treatment option to them, again, under the clinical trial framework that we have discussed.

Dr. JONES. A quick story of frustration of how this can go for patients. In Colorado, Colorado Blue Cross/Blue Shield indemnity insurance will pay for this procedure. Colorado also enforces or deals with the policy issues for Federal employees and Federal employee Blue Cross will not pay in the State of Colorado for these issues.

Colorado Blue Cross/Blue Shield offers an HMO which is alleged to have the same scientific panel as the indemnity insurance company or many of the same individuals. And both the indemnity company and the HMO's say they make their decisions based on best scientific evidence yet the indemnity company reimburses. The HMO does not.

Mr. MYERS. Everybody admitted the only people admitted in the ABMT therapy are those in the clinical trial study. How does one get into that if you are not a Federal employee? I know it is almost impossible if you are a Federal employee. Who approves this? Who is the clearinghouse?

Dr. CHAMPLIN. I think we may have discussed this while you were making your vote. There are a range of things that fall under what is clinical trial. There is Phase I and II clinical trials that involve patients in certain categories getting new treatments or assessment of the efficacy of a change in the basic treatment again with the hope that it would improve the outcome. And so a patient would not need to be randomized or have the coin flip to determine if they can get the transplant or not in such a study.

These types of treatments are widely available and it is possible for most patients to participate in those types of trials. And all of the speakers have urged that patients would be getting marrow transplants, be participating in those studies, that we can get information from them that can help us in defining the role for this treatment and in what patients it is useful and what patients it is not. So we would, again, encourage people to participate in those studies and it should be available to almost anyone.

The limitation is usually on the insurance company supporting a patient's access to those studies. And I have had the frustrating situation with some Blue Cross patients that the Blue Cross company would say we don't pay for clinical research so you can treat that patient but you can't put them on a clinical trial. You can use exactly the same treatment, but they can't be registered or analyzed as part of a clinical study, which is lunacy.

Mr. MYERS. Then it appears the patient would have to leave their oncologist if they are out in a small community or someplace and go into one of the approved treatment centers approved by NCI. Is that what you're saying?

Dr. CHAMPLIN. Most community oncologists, fortunately for the patients, don't attempt to administer treatments of this type that require——

Mr. MYERS. Didn't we have different——

Dr. CHAMPLIN. Pardon?

Mr. MYERS. I am sorry for interrupting you. We had the testimony the treatment was given in unapproved centers. I don't know where they are. We didn't get into that, at least not when I was here.

Dr. CHAMPLIN. One of my concerns, and also of the other speakers——

Mr. MYERS. Podunk hospital does it.

Dr. CHAMPLIN. Podunk hospital, yes. The individuals at small community hospitals with no training in giving intensive doses of chemotherapy or in doing transplantation procedures are trying to do this without the proper experience, training and without the institutional oversight that is present in a large academic center or even large city hospitals where they have a group of individuals, the institutional review boards that are knowledgeable in cancer treatment that can review the program and make sure that ethical, effective and safe treatments are being conducted and that clinical research studies are feasible and proper that are being done.

So we see that is an attempt to move technology, perhaps prematurely, to a community setting in the center that cannot give a treatment safely or effectively is being done, and we have concern for the benefit of the patients that would be participating in that type of treatment.

Mr. MYERS. Well, now, there have been other treatments, other therapies that have been found to be more successful other than the standard chemotherapy treatment, such as the thermally enhanced radiation, which is California's Loma Linda, there is one I think in Boston, now possibly in Texas where I think the University of Texas may have one in the future where the lineac creates a higher radiation burn but is able to define it and only hit the tumor and not do damage to other cells around it.

There is, of course, a standard threat in chemotherapy. Some oncologists boost—after a few series, start boosting. My wife had, after about two months of treatments, they started increasing each time 10 percent. I don't remember which chemicals were increased. Over a 14-month period, what she was taking very, very powerful. She was very able to tolerate it without ill-effects other than being bald and a few things like that, no ill effects from it and, without surgery, her breast cancer was nine centimeters when it was first discovered. You could feel a little scar tissue, but it was done because it was enhanced, not thermally, but increased by radiation.

Are some of those possibly just as successful as the ABMT, chemo?

Dr. CHAMPLIN. Radiation therapy is a local treatment to the primary breast cancer.

Mr. MYERS. I mix those two.

Dr. CHAMPLIN. In certain patients, it is very effective and can cure the local disease site. The problem with breast cancer is that it is usually a systemic disease, and small numbers of breast cancer cells circulate through the system early in the course of the disease, see that other tissues may recur at some later time in the liver, the bones or the lung and some other tissue and radiating the breast would not address the systemic disease.

So the three options or two options in treating that is hormonal therapies or chemotherapy, and the high dose treatment is a way to give the chemotherapy treatment in the most effective fashion.

Mr. MYERS. Does anyone have any comment about the other, the boosting chemo and enhanced radiation, or a combination of both?

Dr. JONES. I have an indirect comment about that. That is, as I pointed out earlier, one of the frustrations in boosting of chemotherapy with bone marrow transplant has been accepted for other indications and conditions where, certainly, the consensus at my center where we even do these procedures is that the data is not as compelling as it is for breast cancer.

And it is particularly frustrating for patients who see these reimbursements to look at that and say, it seems difficult to define a scientific basis for reimbursement decisions based on these criteria.

Dr. HENDERSON. I think the thing that is important to keep, in my mind, is the fact that if you go to centers all over the world, excellent centers, the programs that are going to be advised in those centers are going to be different and they are going to be unique for those centers. Once something has been proven, unequivocally, then there will be a commonality.

So, for example, throughout the 1970s, and even into the early 1908s, there was a lot of controversy about whether it was worthwhile to give any kind of, either, chemotherapy or hormone therapy right after mastectomy, let's say, or after lumpectomy and radiation, did that have any value of prolonging life? It was the same kind of debate that is going on here.

But, you know, it was a little bit different era. And at that point—and insurance companies often times didn't pay for it as well until the evidence came out. We started doing the first trials of vagomin chemotherapy in 1958. In 1979, the NIH had a consensus conference in which they concluded there was unequivocal evidence that chemotherapy, given right after the primary diagnosis, would prolong the lives of premenopausal women. Overnight, that became standard treatment.

I personally thought for example, Tamoxifan, it is a drug, would not have much impact on survival. And in fact most of us on this side of the Atlantic felt that. On the other hand, in Europe, they were prescribing this regularly for postmenopausal women and in fact were able, eventually, to show with trials that this did prolong survival.

When I saw that evidence in a way that was convincing, I changed my practice, literally, overnight, even though that was not the hypothesis I had been working on myself. What I am trying to say, when things are done at one institution or another and there isn't the general applicability, that means the evidence isn't there. That is somebody's theory, that is somebody's experiment, and sometimes that is done and it is called an experiment and sometimes it isn't. I think that was some of the points that had been made by both my colleagues here.

But once it is very clear that something does work, it will change practice. Unfortunately, when we demonstrate that something doesn't work, that does not necessarily change practice.

A classic example is DES. We demonstrated in randomized trials that there was no advantage of giving DES to women who were of high risk of multiple miscarriages. Nonetheless, it was perceived well, we have got to do something, women who had four and five miscarriages and badly wanted a family, and literally thousands of women continue to get DES in the 1950's and 1960's.

That was even after the randomized trials were done. Of course, 20 years later, we paid a fairly high price for that.

Mr. MYERS. You spoke about Tamoxifan. The animal study on Tamoxifan was pretty conclusive, it seemed to me. The study done on rats and guinea pigs and some of the others they have done, the Tamoxifan was very conclusive evidence that it does—not 100 percent. Nothing is 100 percent, I guess.

But anyway, that be as it may, the thing that bothers me here, you testified ABMT should be applied after surgery. Do you take a patient that hasn't had surgery? Do they have to have either a lump or radical to qualify for ABMT therapy?

Dr. CHAMPLIN. Some patients, if they are presented with a metastatic disease, they are treated with chemotherapy as their initial treatment and would not need to have the mastectomy to receive a transplant. Usually we would advise them to have some definitive local therapy for the primary site, which would be the most likely site that they would recur. Lacking such treatment, either a mastectomy and local radiation would usually be advised. We need to look at each case individually.

Mr. MYERS. Your old hospital, M.D. Anderson, was where my wife went to flip a coin about whether she had a lump or radical mastectomy—as much success one way as the other. That is the reason I have the question about after surgery.

All of you talk about treatment after surgery. One thing that disturbed me very much, out in Indiana, when the family physician feels a lump, sends her to a surgeon, everybody is sent to a surgeon instead of an oncologist, to cut that thing out. I thought we were kind of getting away from that now. It doesn't sound like that from your testimony today.

Dr. JONES. I think there are important studies going on around to address this issue to see whether it is useful for significant types of patients, particularly those with larger tumor masses.

I came back to the thought that all of the women who were here this morning, I believe, participated in trials or studies of various kinds of treatment. Not only do they get good treatment, but we got evidence. I think Dr. Henderson would agree, we are working on the issue of using chemotherapy before the mastectomy, and the data is accumulating but we don't know the answer yet.

Dr. HENDERSON. I do think, though, that even in those settings, the major studies that are going on all involve some sort of surgery. Thus far, no one has abandoned surgery. What they've abandoned is big surgery versus little surgery. But almost everybody gets some form of surgery. There is a relatively small group, maybe 2, 3, 4 percent of patients who never have any surgery whatsoever.

Mr. MYERS. I wouldn't want to go to his hospital. Only problem I have with that——

Dr. HENDERSON. Surgery doesn't necessarily mean mastectomy. It may mean only removing the lump.

Mr. MYERS. I know it is a therapy. Surgeons only get paid if they cut. I had a good friend who was a surgeon. He said to me, "Don't go on a sole recommendation of a surgeon". He said, "We don't get paid unless we cut."

Dr. HENDERSON. They get paid more the more they cut.

Mr. MYERS. You use the word "cure" only in testicular. Is that the only cancer to be cured today. Do you consider these other ladies back here not cured, only in remission?

Dr. CHAMPLIN. Cured is a retrospective term. If you try to rigorously apply it, it means a patient has gone on to live a normal life and died from other causes. Breast cancer is a disease that can recur 20 years later and so that in all of the studies that we have talked with shorter follow-up time than that, one can be hopeful that the patients will be cured.

And I personally believe, based on transplant studies and other situation that is the people in the Stage II group that have been treated and are showing what appears to be a plateau on their survival curve that many of them in fact are cured and that their cure action will improve, but we need longer follow up to know for sure.

Dr. JONES. Breast cancer is a heterogenous disease with respect to when it shows up. But women who get bone marrow transplants, at least at our institution, have a median age of 42 years old. I think in order to definitively prove cure, we will have to follow many of those patients throughout their natural lifetime.

So in order to apply the word cure to them, the studies will probably take at least 30 or 40 years of duration. I think if you are curing, whether we need to wait that long in view of the available data, I would come down on the side that 40 years is too long to wait to decide about this issue, and we can draw conclusions about whether the tumor has disappeared for prolonged periods of time.

Certainly I am persuaded with the data, with respect to bone marrow transplant, there are many more women free of tumor at this time than I would have expected with standard therapy.

Dr. HENDERSON. That is one of the advantages of a randomized trial. You can answer these questions very quickly. For example, the first randomized was in 1948 looking at tuberculosis, early anti-tuberculosis trial. It was clear-cut results, and streptomycin became a major treatment.

It doesn't have to be large. It depends on the disease, the end points. It varies a lot. A randomized trial, you're comparing two outcomes where it has been determined by chance alone that the patient would get one or the other. So you are not trying to wait for years in order to see an outcome compared to some other group until you have waited till the last point in time.

Mr. MYERS. Is it too early—this is my last question.

Is it too early to start talking about the recurrence in those patients who have received ABMT therapy? What is the history of recurrence? Or what is your knowledge of this?

Dr. CHAMPLIN. Some of them will recur. They usually recur at the sites where the disease had been previously. So if they had previously had disease in their liver and they get a response, it would usually come back at the site where the disease was.

So it would indicate that one has not killed all of the clonogenic tumor cells that could possibly grow back, and so we are looking at ways that we could kill that fraction that might have survived the high dose therapy by a number of potential means.

Mr. MYERS. The cancer cell can metastasize to the liver, the same cells?

Dr. CHAMPLIN. The ones that went to the liver, you presumably didn't kill them all.

Mr. MYERS. It is a cancer cell in the liver.

Dr. CHAMPLIN. That if somebody had breast cancer and it spreads to their liver——

Mr. MYERS. There are different kinds of cancer.

Dr. CHAMPLIN. It is the breast cancer. It started in the breast, spread to other parts of their body, and then you treat it, it shrinks. If you shrink it enough that you can't detect it by any X-ray or standard test, it is called a remission.

If the patients relapse, they tend to relapse in areas where they have had the disease before, and it is the same tumor when you biopsy that site again.

Mr. MYERS. I apologize. My wife had breast cancer, started 14 months of chemo, two months later she had secondary stages of cervical cancer. Entirely different cancer. Breast cancer metastasized to the cervix. Two different cancers. That is what I am trying to find out, if it was the same cancer.

Dr. CHAMPLIN. That would be a different cancer cell. The people who have one cancer are statistically more likely to get a second cancer, and there may be genetic predisposition in some people. It may be bad luck in other people.

Mr. MYERS. I guess a person who had appendicitis couldn't get appendicitis but a person who has cancer could get it again.

Dr. CHAMPLIN. Yes, could get another cancer in another tissue.

Mr. MYERS. The thing that we are looking for is how are we going to get these people treated and cured. That is what I am trying to find out, if this is the right way to go about it. Then we ought to give everyone the opportunity to have these.

Dr. CHAMPLIN. How you are going to get more people cured is to continue to support clinical research that would lead to improved therapies. I think all of our concerns as we look at health care reform, where does clinical research come in?

If we are dealing with a situation where we are having managed competition and the cheapest vendor will win in terms of getting contracts, then nobody can do research because no one's supporting the cost of that research.

Mr. MYERS. Wearing another hat with appropriations when we have NCI and NIH come before us, we are looking at two tracts, first, better cure, better treatment, diagnose particular work as well as treatment. The other track is: How can we prevent it?

So where do we put the dollars that we have? What is the better place to spend it. I ask the question. I don't want to take time in this debate. That is different.

Dr. CHAMPLIN. You fund the most meritorious research, whether in basic science or clinical medicine.

Mr. MYERS. Thank you very much for your testimony.

Ms. NORTON. Thank you very much, Mr. Myers. You have, I think, been appropriately frank in bringing some humility to the imperfection of the processes available, even to scientists. And I don't envy what kind of judgment you have to have. These are human procedures, human judgments, and we recognize that.

All things considered, considering all the imperfections, and considering the costs on every side of this question, can it at least be said that reimbursement by an insurance company today, in its judgment, all factors considered, is not inappropriate? Can we get agreement on that?

Dr. HENDERSON. I'm not certain that I understand the question.

Dr. JONES. I didn't understand your question, either.

Ms. NORTON. Considering all the factors that must go into the judgment of an insurance company, some of them medical, some of them legal, some of them commercial, some of them scientific, can we at least get agreement that it is not inappropriate for an insurance company to reimburse for the cost of this treatment?

Dr. CHAMPLIN. As far as for breast cancer in appropriate situations participating in a clinical trial of some type.

Ms. NORTON. Yes. That I could say it is an appropriate thing, that those should be covered.

Ms. NORTON. Dr. Jones?

Dr. JONES. Yes, I believe it is appropriate.

Ms. NORTON. Dr. Henderson?

Dr. HENDERSON. I happen to believe in pluralism, that some people might come to different conclusions. Ideally, we want to get areas of consensus. If you're implying by that statement that the government should tell insurance companies that they——

Ms. NORTON. No, I am not.

Dr. HENDERSON. I wouldn't go that far.

Ms. NORTON. I am talking about the judgment that an insurance company has to make.

Dr. HENDERSON. I like to believe that different doctors—different groups of people can come to different conclusions on most of the things we deal with in life.

Ms. NORTON. That is why I framed it the way I did. Not that they have to do it. Considering—that this is why I put into my equation commercial, legal, medical, and I am just trying to understand whether, in your judgment—I understand that these are judgment calls—this would—we could at least say it is not inappropriate for an insurance company.

Dr. HENDERSON. I agree.

Ms. NORTON. Thank you.

Ms. NORTON. We have talked about and I am very respectful of what it takes to show that something in fact, to use the parlance of the street, works. Dr. Henderson testified that it took decades to know that radical mastectomy didn't work any better than some other treatments.

For example, given the fact that to say that a treatment is definitive and effective is to wait decades, that the question you raise, that person has lived as long anyway can't be answered in a few years' time, have you considered what the standard should then be?

I mean, are you prepared to say indeed what Dr. Henderson has said, let's say in 1940, don't do a radical mastectomy, which is the only thing we know to do because 40 years hasn't expired yet. And we can't say that it is—we can't say that it is a cure. You could not say that then.

I am asking you what a physician in 1940 should have done? What an insurance company should have done? Because it was impossible to say then that the radical mastectomy was a cure, and that it would not recur, and that it was effective, and all of the things that you have established as a standard for knowing when we have an effective treatment. Yes.

Dr. HENDERSON. I was trying to make the opposite point from the one that you took from my comments. In other words, I was trying to make the point that, by delaying randomized trials, we actually delay getting the truth and that the problem with the radical mastectomy was that we accepted it widely without testing it.

But by the time we had the tools to test it, which was quite some time of after it was developed, it took another 30 or 40 years for people to open up their mind because they were so convinced.

Ms. NORTON. A very compelling point. I am trying to put mastectomy in the place that this treatment is now and to ask what should, at that point, let us say, 50 years ago, assuming randomized trials were going on and it would take 40 years to show that in fact it was effective, what should an insurance company have done in 1940?

Dr. HENDERSON. Well, I think she should have done what they are doing with bone marrow transplant now. We are talking about a different era. We are talking about the era before we brought in randomized trials. It is difficult to go back once something is established. That is why—Dr. Jones made the point that most things that are part of standard medicine would not—have not ever been demonstrated by randomized trials to be worthwhile.

It is also quite plausible that a large part of all of what we pay for in medical care doesn't achieve the two ends of medicine, either to make patients live better or live longer or both.

Ms. NORTON. That is precisely my question. Given the fact that you cannot know, what should an insurance company do? What should a doctor do?

Dr. HENDERSON. You can't go back. In other words, what people are trying to do today, I think, researchers, people in policy and so on are saying okay, let's draw a line. We can't go back and retest everything that has ever been developed but we are going to have to have some reasonable way to get answers.

And I would contend—for example, I have been part of this process since 1974 with bone marrow transplant. And I would contend that if we had started the studies, the randomized trials in 1985, which is about the earliest that we could have done them, that we would have answers by now.

That it is sort of an irony because, on the one hand, I don't believe we would ever have done the randomized trials that we are now doing if the insurers had not drawn a line in the sand and say we are going to stop here. On the other hand, I think we would have gotten a lot of the research done a lot faster if insurers had supported trials at a much earlier stage.

I think what has happened in the last three or four years, we have moved from these two ends, from either paying for everything or paying from nothing, to try to begin to define some middle ground. And I am suggesting, and I think all three of us are suggesting, we have to define a fairly large middle ground and much more rapidly.

But this does not mean we have to wait decades. I think we could answer these questions before they appear in the press, before they create hope—in many cases, false hopes—in the minds of the public.

Dr. CHAMPLIN. It is important to keep in mind that randomized trials answer a question—is a treatment better than another treatment that are being studied. During the course of a trial being conducted, at the end of the study, there usually is a new question, at least on your mind. There is what appears to be yet another advance in the field that is continuing to advance during the course of that trial.

So what I expect to happen is, in three years, when the randomized trials are available, we will see that, at least for some patients, the high dose treatment is beneficial. And then there will be yet other studies that would be initiated to try and better address their needs as well as to address the needs of patients that aren't being well served by that particular regimen, so this will be a fluid and moving target. But the randomized trials are important to define the base line of those studies.

Dr. JONES. Insurers have traditionally had this black and white that has been alluded to. If it is research, I am not going to pay for it no matter how meritorious. If it is standard therapy, I will pay for it anyway.

I think what insurance companies should have done in 1940 with the radical mastectomy is to say there is value to research, there are different kinds of mastectomys, we should ask questions and those things should be reimbursed in centers where the questions are being asked. And if they are being done on an ad hoc basis outside of those areas, since we don't know the answer, they shouldn't be reimbursed unless those answers are forthcoming.

There are plenty of variety of trials of bone marrow transplants—not only the coin flip trials, but others—that seek a variety and insurers should value those because, ultimately, it is in their best interest to have those answers.

Had we started the breast cancer trials in 1986, the mortality rate of the major chemotherapy regiment was 86 percent. Today it is 3.5 percent. The cost of the treatment in 1986, even at that time, was $150,000 per patient. Now, ignoring inflation, the typical cost at the University of Colorado is $110,000. So there has been a substantial reduction in cost.

All of those came about because there were a variety of trials to answer or to ask questions and we were getting answers to those. I want OPM to consider the value of that and consider that there is a significant weight of evidence to suggest that the research is not only meritorious but patients may have better outcomes as a result of getting access to these treatments.

Ms. NORTON. So only the coin flip, instead of confining themselves to only the most rigorous trials, the coin flip.

Dr. JONES. Yes. I think I am much more comfortable with making a case there should be access to a broad variety of trials and certainly physicians are much more comfortable with the ideas that they have those options.

I think Dr. Henderson may argue that that would retard the completion of these coin flip trials. But to me the price is too high where one is forced to enter a trial where they don't want a particular option as a price for possibly getting action to the other arm.

Ms. NORTON. This is the question I want to leave you with. It is my last question. Because, in a real sense, you have come head on with competing values in this society, and lawyers greet them all the time, but they are most often not life and death so we sort them out analytically and pat ourselves on the back. You have a much more serious and difficult situation.

We are going to be hearing testimony very soon from an attorney that suggests that a good number of countries' top medical institutions refuse to participate in NCI trials because they believe that the HDC treatment is superior to conventional treatment and that randomized trials, under these circumstances, are unethical. Increasing—here are physicians who obviously understand the methodology, the importance of randomized trials.

I would like for all three of you to comment on that notion and that conclusion of reputable institutions and physicians.

Dr. JONES. For myself, I have trouble with the issue that the trials are unethical per primum because I think, at least in my view, there is no absolutely definitive evidence as to which of the approaches is better, though I believe the preponderance of the evidence favors the high dose approach at this time.

I think, one, I certainly have more trouble if one takes the concept of a randomized trial and then says I am sorry, the only way that you can get access to your doctor's preferred treatment is if you participate in this coin flip. I don't know whether it is unethical, but I know that members of the ethics panel at my hospital have questioned the ethics of this, so that at least it is certainly a matter that I am more comfortable with having as a subject of debate.

Dr. CHAMPLIN. I personally would challenge the thought that the leaders in the field of breast cancer would question the value or the ethical nature of those trials. I think even the most enthusiastic transplant specialist welcomes the completion of these trials to really clarify the role of marrow transplants versus other therapies. And to my knowledge every major authority in the field feels that same way.

Dr. HENDERSON. I have been sitting here thinking, what institutions could this lawyer be bringing up? And the only thing that I can come up with is either they are institutions that I don't have much association with or the other possibility, as I have mentioned before, is that institutions that have many people in them and that doesn't mean that they speak as one voice.

Recently a patient from my own institution came to see me who had previously seen one of the transplanters, and the patient told me that these were the things that she had understood she had heard. And when I picked up the note, which was written by one of the young physicians who was part of that, it was quite consistent with what she was telling me.

I wouldn't consider that either the policy of the University of California, San Francisco and certainly as head of the breast unit, I wouldn't consider that the policy or as head of the whole division. The way I dealt with that was making certain only that the physician brought the patient back and made certain that all the facts were clear in her head. But I was quite willing to allow a physician working in my institution and under my jurisdiction to have a difference of opinion as long as the actual facts and data were correct in the patient's head.

So, you know, you may get spokesmen from any institution who will say one thing or another, but I can't think of a leading expert in breast cancer who is head of a breast cancer service at a major cancer institute in this country who would say that it is unethical to do randomized trials at this point.

Ms. NORTON. Let me thank you for your testimony because it has been very important and very useful. What I fear most for what is going on now is that we are beginning to have members of our profession get into the act. They are too much into your business as it is. I happen to be one of those lawyers who strongly favors tort reform, I believe that people practice preventative medicine—I am sorry, defensive medicine precisely because lawyers are looking to sue anything that moves.

But I have to say to you, I think that unless the profession straightens out this notion of when a patient is entitled to treatment at what stage that litigation is going to loom larger, and I would hate to see litigation destroy or threaten the important value of randomized trials because we have been too narrow in understanding what society requires now.

I am actually heartened by the possibility, at least, I think Dr. Henderson himself said that there is an emerging middle ground. I am heartened by the notion that physicians and scientists are aware of this profound difficulty and that you are trying to work it out. Good luck to you. I am sure the lawyers will be of no assistance.

Thank you very, very much for your very, very important testimony.

Mr. HENDERSON. Thank you.

Ms. NORTON. And finally, I would like to call and thank the last panel, panel five. I would like to apologize to you as well. We certainly had no intention of going on this long. Perhaps you can see by the nature of the testimony, the excellence of the responses which require cross examination, which you certainly understand better than most, why we have gone on so long. You have my profound apologies.

I am inviting Ms. Arlene Gilbert Groch, Esquire; Mr. Richard Carter, Esquire; and Ms. Kim Calder, Director of Public Policy, Cancer Care.

Now, what I would like to do is to finish this testimony—we have been here since 10:00 a.m.—by 3:00 p.m., I would like us to be finished if we could. If I can't, then I won't, because it is most important to hear this. It is as important to hear your testimony as to hear all that has gone before you.

Again, my apologies and my thanks. You can proceed in any order you desire.

STATEMENTS OF ARLENE GILBERT GROCH, ESQUIRE; RICHARD CARTER, ESQUIRE, HUDGINS, CARTER & COLEMAN; AND KIM CALDER, DIRECTOR OF PUBLIC POLICY, CANCER CARE INC.

Ms. GROCH. All right. Thank you.

I am sure you will be happy to hear that I am not going to read a single word from my prepared statement. What I would like to do is address an issue that I think has not been addressed at all today or only minimally. It was raised partially by Ms. McCarty.

OPM has known, pretty much acknowledged since as early as 1991, that ABMT for breast cancer was at least as good as standard therapy. The way they—when done in academic centers, when done in good—under good circumstances. The way they acknowledged it was by changing the contracts which they approved.

Prior to 1991, the insurers and OPM sought to reject this treatment on the grounds that it was investigational or experimental. They won for several years. In 1990, 1991, and most certainly by 1992, they consistently lost that argument. When judges, listening to the testimony of experts on both sides, weighed the evidence presented in an adversarial setting, the courts consistently and almost unanimously came down to the conclusion that it was not experimental, it was not investigational, and therefore could not be excluded under the contracts.

And OPM frequently in 1990, 1991, and even in 1992, ordered Blue Cross, Mail Handlers, et cetera, to pay for the treatment, to provide coverage in settlements because OPM acknowledged, as did the insurers, that they would lose when a de novo review was held by a court.

What has happened is that Ms. McCarty and others like her lost their cases in court because—not because the treatment, the medical issues went against them. Not because the medical evidence was no longer persuasive. To the contrary, it was even more persuasive. But because OPM, in working with the insurance industry, has basically abused the clear language of the FEHBP statute and the congressional regulations passed pursuant therefore.

There are three specific sections that I believe are being abused by OPM in order to deny insureds access to judicial review, to effective judicial review. What OPM is seeking to do—and this goes beyond breast cancer, beyond ABMT.

This is a method by which, I believe, that one of the reasons that they have stuck with this issue, this denial of coverage for breast cancer, for all of these years is because they want to use this issue to obtain total control over the insurance granting or denial of benefits so that, by misinterpreting the statute and misinterpreting the regs, they are trying to obtain a judicial deference standard of review, an arbitrary and capricious standard of review, as opposed to, of course, the reasonable expectations of the insured standard of review, which is not only case law in almost every state in this country, but is also contained in the contract between the insurance companies and OPM as an appendix, called Appendix DB2, which says that an insurance—the insurance contracts must be clear and unambiguous.

What OPM is doing is they are saying Section 890.105 of the regs, which says an insured may seek review from OPM from an insurance denial by the company, to say that that statute doesn't mean may, it means shall. And it doesn't mean the insured has a right of review. It means the insurer also has a right of review.

When Ms. McCarty said much earlier today that she was—she lost her case because she had to go to OPM for review and then the court didn't look at her contract—her issue clearly, she was wrong and some courts have accepted that argument. They are starting, I think, to change now. But what OPM is saying is that that section of the statute is mandatory administrative review. And because it is mandatory administrative review, when OPM then puts its stamp of approval invariably on the side of the insurance company, that is now a final review by an administrative agency and therefore is entitled to deference by the courts?

If OPM succeeds in its endeavor, no insured who has been denied review will be able to get a judicial review. And that, as I say, cuts across every disease, every denial. It gives total control to the insurance company.

The final method by which OPM is seeking to obtain—to limit judicial review is by limiting the access to the courts across the country by saying—by taking the position that every denial of benefits may only be heard in Federal courts. That, in spite of the fact, that Section 5 U.S. Code 8912, the jurisdictional section, specifically says that there is original jurisdiction in the Federal district courts for claims against the United States.

And the reg, Section 890.107 says benefit disputes are not claims against the United States. Benefit claims, even approvals or disapprovals by OPM, are not actions again challenging the legality of the statute.

And so they have twisted these two—three sections to try to change the entire judicial review system for all Federal employees and Federal retirees and to switch the burden of proof from the insurance company to prove that the exclusion is clear and unambiguous to the insured to prove exactly the opposite.

This is going to have a drastic effect, devastating effect. And it is going to give the insurance companies power that this Congress never gave them. And I would ask this commission—this committee to address that broader issue ultimately, as well as the one, the element of that which you have tackled today.

Thank you.

Ms. NORTON. Thank you very much.

[The prepared statement of Ms. Groch follows:]

PREPARED STATEMENT OF ARLENE GILBERT GROCH, ESQUIRE

I am a trial attorney who, during the past eighteen months, has represented women throughout the country who needed coverage from their federal employee insurance policy and other insurers for HDC/ABMT for treatment of breast cancer. In each Federal Employee Health Benefits Act (FEHBA) case I handled, the Office of Personnel Management (OPM) adamantly supported the insurance industry against the federal employee.

OPM has elected to submit women with breast cancer to a standard which has never been applied to any other group, and which is medically and legally indefensible. (See attached 31 statements from Professors of Medicine and Department Chiefs at such institutions as Harvard Medical School, MD Anderson, Yale University, Dana-Farber Cancer Institute, etc. affirming that HDC/ABMT has been their treatment of choice for certain breast cancer patients for the past several years. See also attached summary of the relevant case law in which nearly every state and federal judge who has considered the medical evidence in adversarial, do novo judicial reviews, has rejected the "investigative" defense espoused here by OPM.)

Perhaps the most eloquent testimony was offered in a 1991 deposition by Dr. Christopher F. Sirridge, M.D., then Assistant Professor of Medicine at the University of Missouri-Kansas City, Department of Hematology and Oncology.

[If] my wife or your daughter had [breast cancer * * *] I would look them straight in the eye and tell them an autologous bone marrow transplantation with high dose chemotherapy gives them the best change of a disease-free survival, potential cure and overall survival advantage. It would be unconscionable to look at a patient, as well as a relative or a wife or daughter, regardless of my emotional ties and not offer this as a potential treatment.

I doubt if any NCI, OPM, or Blue Cross Blue Shield executive would reject HDC/ABMT for themselves, their wives or their daughters, if they were in the position of my clients and other similarly situated women.

The position of OPM is: (1) inconsistent with the overwhelming weight of reliable medical/scientific data; (2) adverse to the medical and financial interests of federal employees and retirees; (3) non-responsive to the concern of most Members of Congress and the mood of the country as expressed in the letter from Congresswomen Holmes, Schroeder and approximately 56 other Members; and (4) contradictory to the expressed goals of President and Mrs. Clinton to eliminate gender bias in the provision of health benefits and to reduce the death toll (46,000 women per year) from breast cancer. As Mrs. Clinton said, "Women have been shortchanged * * * in very graphic ways" under current federal health care policy. Breast cancer was specifically identified by her as a health concern for which women do not receive enough money and attention from the federal government. [The Press, Atlantic City, NJ, 2/24/93]

OPM relies on the insurance industry funded NCI studies to delay having to accept the reality that HDC/ABMT is the state of the art treatment for some of the approximately 15,000 women per year who are appropriate candidates for the treatment. (Group Practice Managed Health Care News, April, 1993). This financial relationship and rationale are both eerily reminiscent of the cigarette-industry and its industry funded so-called independent research studies which, for decades, they have used to justify continuing to sell cigarettes on the claim that there is "no conclusive evidence" that cigarette smoking contributes to cancer. Stranger bedfellows, indeed, for this administration whose goal is quality health care through affordable insurance for all.

In the process of litigating these cases I have learned some very disturbing facts about the symbiotic relationship between OPM and the carriers:

1. OPM purports to be acting as agent for all federal employees, negotiating on their behalf with the carriers. yet OPM has negotiated a contract which requires the employees [through the premiums they pay into the national insurance fund] to pay part of the carrier's legal fees when the employees have to sue to collect their benefits. Meanwhile, the employee/retiree has to pay not only her/his own legal fees but also to contribute to those of their insurer! The remainder of the insurer's legal fees are paid by the taxpayers, through the federal government's contribution to the fund. Whose interest was OPM protecting when it negotiated that contract provision?

2. The carriers have routinely denied payment of benefits to women with breast cancer seeking HDC/APCR, while covering it for other diseases for which no randomized clinical trials have ever been required, and for many of which the results are "unequivocally inferior to those for breast cancer." Submission to the Committee by Dr. Roy Jones.

3. In 1989 and 1990 the carriers argued in court that their denial was justified because HDC/APCR was "experimental" when given to women with breast cancer. After a series of judicial decisions rejecting that rationale and compelling coverage, they changed the terms of their FEHBP contracts and argued that women with breast cancer were denied treatment simply because the terms of the contract excluded them.

4. In these later cases, plaintiffs argue that the carrier has failed to provide adequate notice of the purported exclusion, that the exclusion is too vague and ambiguous to be enforceable, and that the exclusion of this medically appropriate and necessary treatment violates the Americans With Disabilities Act, the Equal Employment Opportunities Act, and the Equal Pay Act. The carriers respond that they are merely complying with the mandate of OPM. They also make it as difficult as possible for insureds to obtain meaningful judicial review by (a) seeking to limit access to the courts by trying to remove all cases to the federal courts, (b) demanding that the insured exhaust her administrative [but patently futile] option review to OPM, even though OPM admits it does not review the medical needs of the patient relying instead upon its interpretation of the contract, (c) seeking to impose an "arbitrary and capricious" standard of review giving total deference to the rubber stamp review by OPM, and (d) by raising other complex issues of federal jurisdiction, preemption, conflict of laws, etc.

What is the result of the "leadership" of OPM and the federal insurers in continuing to fight these sick women in the courts long after medical science has concurred that this treatment will increase their chance for a 5-year relapse free survival by 15% to 35% over "conventional" treatment?

One result is that the factors deciding this life and death issue of access to medical treatment are the patient's wealth, education, connections, and therefore her ability to find and hire an attorney willing and able to take on adversaries such as the Blue Cross Blue Shield Association and the federal government—and to do so in a case with little hope of appropriate compensation. Then she must be able to maintain her health long enough to prevail in her David v. Goliath legal battle against two incredible powerful and wealthy adversaries, while simultaneously fighting her cancer.

As the Duke study published in February 1994 proved, a woman's medical condition is not a factor in insurers' decisions. Nor is it a factor relevant to either OPM or the federal insurers. These women then become divided into the following categories:

1. The vast majority of women are too sick, too poor, too uneducated, and/or otherwise unable to retain legal counsel to challenge the carrier's initial denial. These women die.

2. A few women manage to hire attorneys and file suit to compel coverage. The carriers will promise coverage to some of them, mainly through settlement agreements with secrecy clauses. Even fewer will get the treatment that might have saved their lives.

A. Some carriers settle out-of-court fairly readily when counsel intervenes, and agree to provide those few women with treatment.

B. When women get a favorable decision or appear about to do so the carrier often offers to pay for the treatment and not appeal the adverse decision, on the condition that the woman ask the court not to enter the decision of record, or to vacate it. Most women, faced with the possibility of leaving their family not only motherless but impoverished as well if the carrier successfully appeals the trial court's decision, have little choice but to accept that offer. Thus the insurers limit the number of recorded and/or appellate decisions favoring plaintiffs.

C. In other cases the carriers prevail because the plaintiff's attorney is unprepared either because of time constraints [these cases must, of necessity, be handled on an extremely expedited basis] or because of inexperience. Many women are represented by lawyers who are trying valiantly to help because they are a friend or family member, but who have little experience dealing with the complex federal jurisdiction and substantive issues raised by the carriers.

To compound the injustice, many of those women who are ultimately successful in using the courts to compel coverage, later learn to their dismay that by the time they have succeeded legally, they have lost medically. All too often their cancer has spread so much while the insurer delayed providing an answer to their request for precertification and during the litigation battle that followed, their cancer spread so much that they were no longer medically able to benefit from the treatment. Their window of opportunity for life (or at least for an improved quality of life) had been slammed shut.

OPM has used the breast cancer issue to try to establish a precedent in which every insurer's denials of any benefit (not only HDC/ABMT) will be immune from *de novo* judicial review. If OPM succeeds, the federal insurance companies will win in court nearly every time an insured has the temerity to challenge their denials of benefits. Under the OPM/Blue Cross plan, an insured employee or retiree could only prevail if no reasonable explanation or justification could be dreamt up (even in hindsight) for the denial, simply because, in almost every case, its benefit denial had been rubber stamped by OPM.

I ask this Committee to examine the motivation of OPM to maintain such a medically and ethically unsound position. Why does OPM aid, abet, encourage, and spend taxpayer and employee dollars to promote such a policy? Why has OPM allowed Blue Cross to waste taxpayer and federal employee/retiree dollars as was demonstrated by the hearings held last week by Senator Nunn? One reason may be the revolving door policy between OPM and the federal insurance providers. Hopefully, the relationship between OPM and those it is mandated to regulate will continue to be explored by this and other committees in future hearings.

Thank you for giving me the opportunity to present the viewpoint of the women who have had to fight this battle alone, one at a time, against such unfair odds.

SUMMARIES OF OPINIONS OF MEDICAL EXPERTS

The issue: Does the "reliable clinical evidence" indicate [. . .] That HDC/ABMT is at least as effective as conventional treatment for breast cancer and is worth the added risk?

The answer: "High-Dose Chemotherapy and BMT has emerged as the most potent treatment yet developed for advanced or high-risk breast cancer." "Breast cancer has now become the disease most frequently treated with BMT in the United States." Dr. Roy Jones, M.D., Ph.D. Top scientists and medical directors at most of the major teaching hospitals in this country agree with him.

LETTERS DEMONSTRATING THE CONSENSUS OF MEDICAL OPINION FROM 1988 TO 1990

1. 1988—MD Anderson Cancer Center, Dr. Gabriel N. Hortobagyi, M.D., Professor of Medicine, Chief, Breast Medical Oncology, and Gary Spitzer, M.D., Deputy Dir., Bone Marrow Transplantation and Professor of Medicine.

Third party payers in our area have in general recognized that the results of high dose chemotherapy with autologous bone marrow reinfusion are not only appropriate therapy but offer a higher likelihood of response than previously utilized standard treatments.

2. 1988—University of California, Los Angeles, David Golde, M.D., Professor and Chief, Division of Hematology-Oncology.

Autologous transplantation in breast cancer has, as you know, met with moderate success already and I do not consider it as being experimental therapy. At UCLA we have quite an active autologous bone marrow transplant program for solid tumors.

3. 1988—Michigan Transplant, the U. of Michigan Organ Transplantation Center, Medical Director, Bone Marrow Transplant Program.

The term "experimental" is a term that is all too frequently used for therapies that can be useful for the treatment of patients. It appears that there is a large gap between experimental therapies and standard therapies. It is our concern here at the University of Michigan that it is required that a therapy be shown to be "curative" before it is moved from the experimental category to the standard category. However, as you and I and everyone else in medicine are aware these therapies can be of use in our constant battle against malignant disease even when not curative. Though our goal is to cure these diseases, there are actually very few diseases in medicine that are curable but rather are chronic diseases that we attempt to control. In sustaining a reasonable quality of life, a period of time whether it is a few months to a few years, is the goal of therapy [. . .] we believe that the chance for cure in this disease by autologous bone marrow transplantation today is real.

4. 1988—Kendall Cancer Center, Miami, Florida, Charles Vogel, M.D. F.A.C.P., Medical Director.

While I am a strong proponent of palliative therapies in the management of most patients with metastatic breast cancer, I am fully in favor of autologous bone marrow rescue programs for selected subsets of patients. While it is true that we will gain information from all such patients entered into such programs, I would not consider this truly investigational.

5. 1988—University of Wisconsin, Clinical Cancer Center, Douglass C. Tormey, M.D., Ph.D., Professor, Departments of Human Oncology and Medicine.

We are certainly performing this procedure here in high risk adjuvant patients and in stage 4 patients. It is my belief that this is one of the therapeutic approaches available to these patients and in many instances is the most efficacious approach.

6. 1988—Medical College of Virginia, Virginia Commonwealth University, I. David Goldman, M.D., Chairman, Division of Hematology/Oncology, Director, Massey Cancer Center.

Craig Howe, Director of our Bone Marrow Transplantation program and I strongly support your position regarding the role of autologous bone marrow transplantation for patients with solid tumors. We are particularly convinced that this modality has an important role in the treatment of patients with breast cancer with low tumor burdens. It is [. . .] currently being covered by government health agencies and the major private carriers.

7. 1988—National Surgical Adjuvant Project for Breast and Bowel Cancers, Pittsburgh, Pennsylvania, Bernard Fisher, M.D.

This therapy is increasing in scope and offers some patients the only chance for an improvement in their life by bringing metastatic disease under control. At this point in time when therapies for cancer are becoming more sophisticated and complex, we can not permit those who might benefit from such therapy to be denied it because of third-party payers' reluctance to support it.

8. 1988—University of Washington, Seattle, Washington, Robert B. Livingston, M.D., Professor of Medicine, Head, Division of Oncology.

(ABMT), is a procedure of proven value in the management of patients with metastatic breast cancer. I would no longer regard the therapy itself as experimental, although the specific components of the treatment regimen which may prove optimal certainly remain to be defined [. . .] . (we have seen one in eight patients treated between 1983 and 1986, [have had durable complete remissions] currently at 40+ months)

9. 1988—Harvard Medical School, Lowell E. Schnipper, M.D., Chief, Oncology Division Beth Israel Hospital.

It has been my contention that this treatment modality, for appropriately selected patients, represents the best available therapy. A third party payor's refusal to reimburse for this treatment on the basis of it's experimental nature denies the fact that, in selected clinical settings now considered to be incurable, this novel form of therapy will prove to be effective.

10. 1988—The University of Texas, Health Science Center at San Antonio, C. Kent Osborne, M.D., Professor of Medicine.

As you know, there has been a considerable body of research generated with this technique in breast cancer in the past few years. In patients with newly diagnosed advanced breast cancer that is previously untreated, response rates, particularly complete response rates, are among the highest of any treatment regimen recorded to date.

11. 1988—Fox Chase Cancer Center, Robert F. Ozols, M.D., Ph.D., Chairman, Department of Medical Oncology.

It is quite clear in many malignancies including breast cancer and heavily pretreated testicular cancer, that ABMT is capable of inducing a clinically meaningful response. In certain circumstances this appears to be the only form of therapy currently available that has a substantial likelihood of inducing a response and in this situation, I certainly would not characterize autologous bone marrow treatment as experimental.

12. 1088—The University of Michigan Medical School, Allen S. Lichter, M.D., Professor and Chairman, Department of Radiation Oncology.

Current studies indicate that more than 50% of patients with recurrent and resistent solid tumors respond to combinations of high dose chemotherapy with marrow infusion, and approximately 25% of these patients develop a complete response. Diseases that have shown to be responsive to this type of therapy include small cell lung cancer, breast carcinoma, [. . .] For people who have failed standard therapy, ABMT may be the only therapy that offers them the chance of long-term disease free survival, especially when we see younger patients who are otherwise in good health. [. . .] This therapy has been around for many years [. . .] It is far from experimental in the opinion of our group. For third parties to not reimburse for this activity is to deny the results of an enormous body of literature that supports the usefulness of this treatment in select cases.

13. 1988—Yale University, Edwin C. Cadman, M.D., Department of Internal Medicine.

Breast cancer is routinely lethal in all cases; for those who have had bone marrow transplants, their lives have been improved considerably. There are even patients who may have been cured.

14. 1988—Dana-Farber Cancer Institute, Boston, Massachusetts, Emil Frei III, M.D., Director and Physician-in-Chief.

It is established that this approach produces a high complete response rate in patients with metastasic breast cancer. Conservative established treatment is not curable, does not prolong survival and produces at best partial responses in 40%–50% of patients. Thus, autologous bone marrow transplantation represents in my judgment, excellent treatment for the disease.

15. 1989—Lawrence H. Einhorn, M.D., Distinguished Professor of Medicine, Indiana University Medical Center, Indianapolis, Indiana.

Over the past several years, the most important research in this area has been the use of high dose chemotherapy followed by autologous bone marrow transplantation to protect the patient from the effects of this chemotherapy. High does chemotherapy can successfully overcome drug resistance, improve survival, and make this otherwise lethal disease a potentially curable disease. [. . .] I very strongly feel that it would be unethical, if not unconscionable to deny someone care that is felt to be curative when there is no curative alternative for that patient purely because the patient does not have the financial support to cover the cost of the treatment and her insurance company will not provide coverage. I do not view this as experimental therapy but I view it as standard therapy in this situation and this is a belief that is shared by most major cancer researchers and this is a view that is held by most experts in the field of breast cancer in the United States in 1989.

16. 1989—Georgetown University Medical Center, Marc E. Lippman, M.D., Professor of Medicine and Pharmacology, Georgetown University Medical School.

Stated in other words, among all other therapy options known to me, it is my firm medical opinion that ABMT is the optimal therapy. As such, I consider it neither experimental, investigative, or educational in the present circumstances [. . .]

17. 1990—M. John Kennedy, MB, MRCPI, Johns Hopkins Oncology Center.

We have thus far treated 24 women with metastatic breast cancer in this fashion. No patient has died in the hospital and the median length of hospitalization after bone marrow reinfusion is 30 days. Nine patients remain in a stable remission without further therapy. We feel that this therapy offers our patient the single best opportunity for control of her cancer.

18. 1988—Duke University Medical Center, William P. Peters, M.D., Ph.D., Director, Bone Marrow Transplantation Program.

[. . .] in our program [we] have now treated over 150 patients in this setting [. . .] these are results in excess of any currently available regimen for the treatment of metastatic breast cancer.

19. 1989—Duke University Medical Center, Roy B. Jones, M.D., Ph.D., [then] Assistant Professor, Department of Medicine.

[. . .] I have been involved in the treatment of more than 200 patients with breast cancer using high-dose chemotherapy and autologous bone marrow support [. . .]. Standard chemotherapy is essentially totally ineffective in preventing relapse and death from breast cancer in this circumstance [. . .]. The results of this intensive program are so superior to conventional treatment that there is already little question they represent a therapeutic advance. Our treatment program has been reviewed and approved by such bodies as the Cancer and Leukemia Group B, the National Cancer Institute [. . .]. Given the substantial therapeutic benefit which we have already documented for these patients, this treatment is not investigative, mainly for research purposes or experimental in nature. This technique is for therapeutic treatment to the patient. I strongly support the positions of Drs. Yanovich, Howe, and many others across the country who have recognized this as the optimal therapy for this patient.

20. 1989—The Johns Hopkins Oncology Center, Nancy E. Davidson, M.D., Assistant Professor of Oncology.

The intent of the therapy is not for research or investigation. Rather the purpose of the recommended therapy is to treat [Jane Doe's] breast cancer. I believe that no other therapy offers her a better chance for long-term survival.

21. 1988—University of Louisville, Roger H. Herzig, M.D., Marion F. Beard Professor of Hematology, Director, Bone Marrow Transplant Program.

I have been involved in clinical trials of intensive therapy with marrow rescue since 1972 [. . .]. While the optimum preparative regimen has not been found, it is my strong feeling that the procedures involved with this type of therapy are not experimental [. . .]. While studies are being performed to determine better regimens, the underlying concepts of intensive therapy with marrow rescue are well-known and should not be considered experimental. For patients with refractory malignancies, response rates between 40 and 70% are frequently obtained, with 10–20% of patients having durable responses of over a [. . .]. Other responsive tumors have been breast cancer [. . .] for many patients, this approach is the best alternative and may be the only one with curative potential.

22. 1988—Harvard Medical School, Department of Radiation Therapy, Jay R. Harris, M.D. Clinical and Educational Director.

I am writing to you [. . .] to indicate my support for this treatment as standard therapy in selected patients with advanced breast cancer [. . .]. The use of ABMT is an important and credible form of therapy. I can tell you that ABMT is being actively pursued in breast cancer patients both at the Dana Farber Cancer Institute and the Beth Israel Hospital here at Harvard Medical School. I believe it would be highly unfortunate if health insurance carriers did not support ABMT at major cancer centers such as yours.

SWORN CERTIFICATIONS DEMONSTRATING THE CONSENSUS OF MEDICAL OPINION FROM 1991 TO DATE

1. 1991 Christopher F. Sirridge, M.D., Assistant Professor of Medicine at the University of Missouri-Kansas City, Department of Hematology and Oncology. Sworn Testimony given in *White* v. *Caterpillar, Inc.,* (8th Cir.)

[There are] three positive arenas of information and arenas of support that are now available to those oncologists who are interested in the field. The first is that high dose chemotherapy with autologous bone marrow transplant was the first treatment ever to produce substantial numbers of complete responses in breast cancer. [. . .] The second piece of information was that in all studies done there was most definitely an improved three year disease-free survival over those patients treated with conventional therapy. The third piece of valid information is that the toxicity from the procedure itself appeared to be reasonable and well within the gravity of the disease as well as the treatment. Pg. 188, 3–19

I also want to make it quite clear to those in this court that disease free survival is an important, valid and very worthwhile goal in the treatment of a malignancy. Pg. 190, 5–8

[If] my wife or your daughter had [breast cancer . . .] I would look them straight in the eye and tell them an autologous bone marrow transplantation with high dose chemotherapy gives them the best chance of a disease-free survival, potential cure and overall survival advantage. It would be unconscionable to look at a patient, as well as a relative or a wife or daughter, regardless of my emotional ties and not offer this as a potential treatment. Pg. 199, 10–20

2. 1993—University of Colorado Health Sciences Center, Roy B. Jones, Ph.D., M.D.

ABMT treatment is not "investigational" in any generic sense of the term; rather, it is a commonly used technique which has been performed upon thousands of patients having various types of cancer, and several thousand patients with breast cancer. I have performed more than 400 ABMT treatments on patients with breast cancer. The procedure provides patients with a good chance for long term control of their disease. Numerous reports, including literature articles from Duke University, the M.D. Anderson Hospital (Houston, TX), the Dana Farber Cancer Institute (Boston, MA), The Johns Hopkins Medical Center (Baltimore, MD), and the University of Chicago document that between 15% and 30% of the patients undergoing this treatment survive between 3 and 5 years without evidence for tumor recurrence. When patients undergo treatment for Stage IV breast cancer with conventional chemotherapy, the probability of similar relapse-free survival is between 0.3% and 2%, based on large reports from the M.D., Anderson Hospital and the Mayo Clinic.

3. 1994—University of Colorado Health Sciences Center, Roy B. Jones, Ph.D., M.D., testimony before Congress.

The 5-year relapse-free survival for high-risk primary breast cancer treated with BMT is 35% better than any result reported in the medical literature by any research group using any conventional treatment.

4. 1992—University of California, Los Angeles, Stephen D. Nimer, M.D., Acting Director, Bone Marrow Transplant Unit.

I consider the treatment of HDCT–ABMT for breast cancer to be the generally accepted medical practice in our locale.

5. 1992—The Detroit Medical Center, Lyle L. Sensenbrenner, M.D. Director, Bone Marrow Transplantation Program.

We feel that this is the proper therapy for breast cancer and routinely refer patients to a facility that does perform such procedures.

6. 1992—Hematology-Oncology Associates of Columbia, Joseph J. Muscato, M.D., F.A.C.P.

. . . high dose chemotherapy and autologous bone marrow or peripheral stem cell transplant is a necessary and appropriate option in the treatment of breast cancer . . . It is my opinion that this treatment is generally accepted medical practice in our locale.

7. 1992—Bone Marrow Transplant Program, Medical Center of Delaware, R. Bradley Slease, M.D.

Our Cancer Treatment Program at the Medical Center of Delaware provides [HDC/ABMT] for certain stages of Breast Cancer. These procedures are performed under the auspices of the National Cancer Institute's approved protocols.

8. 1992—Albert Einstein Cancer Center, Niculae Ciobanu, M.D.

Many of my colleagues and I do not consider autologous BMT as an experimental form of treatment since we believe there is sufficient literature evidence that high-dose chemotherapy and autologous BMT is clearly superior to any other treatment approach when used in the adjuvant setting and that 10–20% of women with metastatic breast cancer can be placed in long term progression-free status using this high-dose treatment approach.

9. 1992—Tufts University School of Medicine—New England Medical Center, David P. Schenkein, M.D., Assistant Professor of Medicine.

We do offer high dose chemotherapy with autologous bone marrow rescue at our transplant unit for patients with breast cancer.

10. 1992—St. Joseph's Hospital and Medical Center, Bone Marrow Transplantation Program, Paterson, NJ, Arnold D. Rubin, M.D.

Under the appropriate circumstances we consider this generally acceptable medical practice in our area.

11. 1992—The Mount Sinai Medical Center, Director Bone Marrow Transplantation Program, Steven M. Fruchtman, M.D., Assistant Professor of Medicine.

We are one of a number of centers in this geographic area that provides this therapy, and believe it is necessary medical care for these patients.

12. 1992—University of Rochester Medical Center, Jacob M. Rowe, M.D., F.A.C.P., Professor of Medicine, Director of Hematology Clinical Services.

The Bone Marrow Transplant Unit of the University of Rochester Medical Center does indeed provide high dose chemotherapy with autologous stem cell transplant as treatment for certain categories of women with breast cancer.

13. 1992—University of Nevada, School of Medicine, Joao L. Ascensao, M.D., Ph.D., Professor of Medicine, University of Nevada-Reno.

Auto BMT either as adjuvant or treatment for breast cancer is accepted in our community and we believe that it may be cost effective with the recent advance in Biotherapy of cancer.

14. 1992—The Temple University Comprehensive Cancer Center (CCC), Kenneth F. Mangan, M.D., Associate Professor of Medicine, Director, Bone Marrow Transplantation Program.

Our Center provides [HDC/ABMT/APCR] for treatment with women with stage II to IV breast cancer.

15. 1992—The Ohio State University, Peter J. Tutschka, M.D., Professor of Medicine and Pathology.

Such treatment of high dose chemotherapy and autologous bone marrow transplantation for metastatic breast cancer is generally accepted medical practice in our medical community.

16. 1992—The Alta Bates Comprehensive Cancer Center, Jeffrey L. Wolf, M.D.

Our institution is currently providing [HDC/ABMT] for the treatment of both adjuvant and metastatic breast cancer [for] patients with high-risk breast cancer.

17. 1992—Indiana University Hospitals, E. Randolph Broun, M.D., Medical Director, Indiana University/Indiana Regional Cancer Center.

We have treated approximately 40 women in this manner. We certainly feel that for selected women, this represents the treatment of choice.

18. 1992—Roger H. Herzig, M.D., Director, University of Louisville, Bone Marrow Transplant Program.

During the last year, we have treated about 50 women with breast cancer using a dose-intensive therapy approach . . . It is also my opinion that the exclusion on the grounds that such treatment is experimental or investigational is inappropriate. While the best way to treat these women may not be known, I believe the use of dose-intensive therapy with appropriate supportive care is not experimental.

19. 1992—University of California, Los Angeles, Peter J. Rosen, M.D., Professor of Clinical Medicine, Director, Oncology Program.

[HDC/ABMT] for breast cancer has been investigated in the United States and elsewhere during the last decade. Leading medical centers throughout the United States routinely perform this treatment for patients with recurrent (metastatic) breast cancer and in cases of high risk early stage breast cancer as well . . . My feelings with this community suggest strongly to me that this procedure is considered an accepted form of medical practice in the Los Angeles area.

20. 1992—New York Medical College, Tauseef Ahmed, M.D., F.A.C.P., Professor of Medicine, Director of Bone Marrow Transplantation Services.

We have been performing bone marrow transplants at New York Medical College/ Westchester County Medical center since October of 1983 [. . .] Data from several institutions would indicate that marrow transplantation in the setting of breast cancer with ten or more positive nodes as appropriate and reasonable therapy and affords a higher probability of cure than do standard methods of treatment.

I understand the number of Blue Cross/Blue Shield companies would like people to embark on a randomized controlled study. This I find surprising since a control arm is, a) destined to relapse based on historical controls and, b) the study is automatically biased because relapses will get a marrow transplant. This, therefore, does not address the question of whether marrow transplantation is useful, but poses the question whether marrow transplantation should be attempted early or late in these patients.

It is important to note that none of the Blue Cross/Blue Shield companies have ever required a randomized controlled study to compare the efficacy of marrow transplantation in a setting of Hodgkin's disease, nonHodgkin's lymphomas, acute leukemia's or neuroblastoma. Why these companies should be interested in a randomized study appears to stem more from fiscal concerns than the impact of such therapy on the health of the patients that we take care of.

21. 1992—Stanford University Medical Center, Gwynn D. Long, M.D.

We feel that studies published to date suggest that this group of patients with metastatic disease are most likely to benefit from the high dose chemotherapy and marrow rescue.

22. 1992—Marshfield Clinic, Department of Clinical Oncology, Daniel A. Rushing, M.D.

At this time, treatment for recurrent breast carcinoma in our institution is given with curative intent if possible . . . . Based on our own personal experience, as well as that reported in the literature, it appears that treatment is more effective in inducing complete remissions and long-term survivors than is standard-dose chemotherapy. The treatment is given with curative intent, but the word cure cannot be used for any individual patient with breast carcinoma for at least the first five years after treatment.

23. 1992—Tess Artig, R.N. B.S.N., Bone Marrow Transplant Program Manager, University of Utah Medical Center, Division of Hematology/Oncology.

Although conventional therapy does offer some hope, it is found that once a woman recurs with breast cancer, her chance for long-term survival is nil. High-dose chemotherapy followed by peripheral stem cell or autologous marrow rescue may be the only chance for long-term cure and survival.

It is my opinion that financial resources would be better spent in treating these women with recurrent breast cancer rather than having patients fight legal battles.

24. 1992—City of Hope, National Medical Center, Stephen J. Forman, M.D., F.A.C.P., Director.

The fact is that the response rate is higher in patients who therefore benefit from a clinical point of view, particularly in selected patients whose disease is already chemosensitive.

25. 1992—The H. Lee Moffitt Cancer Center at the University of South Florida, Gerald J. Elfenbein, M.D., Professor of Internal Medicine.

We believe that this form of therapy is generally accepted by the medical oncologists of our state as evidenced by the fact that, to date, we have seen 293 women with breast cancer in consultation for this procedure by referral from 114 different physicians.

26. 1992—University of Nebraska Medical Center, Elizabeth C. Reed, M.D., Assistant Professor of Medicine, Clinical Director, Bone Marrow Transplant Unit, Section of Oncology/Hematology.

I can tell you that nearly every oncologist in the state of Nebraska has referred a breast cancer patient for evaluation for transplant and in that sense, I believe the Nebraska oncologists feel that it is an accepted option for the management of breast cancer.

27. Charles M. Strand, M.D., Director, Saint Francis Bone Marrow Transplant Program, Tulsa, Oklahoma.

Since August of 1987, our program has been undertaking both autologous and allogeneic bone marrow transplants for patients with appropriate malignant diseases . . . HDC/ABMT is considered appropriate treatment for young healthy women with otherwise incurable breast cancer, within our medical community in Tulsa, Oklahoma.

28. 1992—Samuel M. Silver, M.D., Ph.D., Director Adult Bone Marrow Transplant Program, University of Michigan.

Sufficient data has accumulated to make us believe that high dose chemotherapy with autologous bone marrow transplantation for metastatic breast cancer which remains sensitive to chemotherapy, is an effective therapy. This therapy is generally accepted medical practice in the State of Michigan and is one of a number of standard therapies for the treatment of this disease.

I enclose with this letter, a position statement from The Michigan Society for Hematology and Oncology on autologous bone marrow transplantation for breast cancer. This states that such treatments have now been established as an effective therapy inducing a number of complete and partial remissions in this disease.

29. 1992—Scripps Clinic and Research Foundation, Robert McMillan, Director, Weingart Center for Bone Marrow Transplantation.

This form of treatment is a generally accepted medical practice in our community for the treatment of certain patients with this disease.

30. 1992—Emory University School of Medicine, W. Ralph Vogler, M.D., Professor of Medicine.

[HDC/ABMT] is effective therapy for certain patients with advanced breast cancer, and is an acceptable medical practice.

31. 1991—William P. Vaughan, M.D., Certified by the American Board of Internal Medicine and Oncology, University of Nebraska Medical Center.

[HDC] treatment supported by bone marrow transplanation is not "investigational" in any common sense meaning of the word. This type of treatment is used commonly on thousands of patients each year. The effectiveness of these procedures is well-established. [. . .]

The fact that approximately 40 different insurance carriers recognize they have a responsibility to reimburse health care providers and patients for this service supports my opinion that this is no longer investigational, but is a clinically and therapeutically useful form of treatment.

SUMMARY OF CASES

The issue: Does "reliable clinical evidence indicate [. . .] That HDC/ABMT is at least as effective as conventional treatment for breast cancer and is worth the added risk?

The answer: Yes, according to nearly every state and federal judge who has considered the testimony of experts from both sides and made a de novo judicial determination on the issue after 1990. The Courts have almost unanimously rejected the "experimental" or "investigational" defense still asserted by OPM to justify denial of treatment. However, OPM acknowledges that the Courts of this land have rejected that claim. Therefore OPM allows the insurers to seek to exclude coverage by specific exclusionary contract language, rather than rely upon their "experimental" or "investigational" claim.

SUMMARY OF CASES IN WHICH THE COURTS MADE A DE NOVO REVIEW OF WHETHER OR NOT HDC/ABMT/APCR IS MEDICALLY NECESSARY AND APPROPRIATE FOR TREATMENT OF BREAST CANCER

A. State cases

Comprecare Insurance Company v. Cynthia Snow, Case No. 92–CV–8087 (Colo. Dist. Ct. Denver Cty. Feb. 16, 1993) (breast cancer; HDC/ABMT; injunction granted after hotly contested hearing as to whether treatment was "experimental")

Miller v. Blue Cross & Blue Shield of N.H., Inc., No. 91–E–411 (Super. Ct. Merrimack County, N.H. Aug. 5, 1991)

Taylor v. Blue Cross and Blue Shield of Michigan, No. 156767 and 156806; LC No. 91–25861, Ct. of Appeals; June 20, 1991, (Stage IV Breast Cancer, HDC/ABMT is not experimental.)

Terninko v. Blue Cross & Blue Shield of N.H. Inc., No. 91–E–517 (1991) (Preliminary injunction compelled coverage under *de novo* standard; case settled before trial)

Valencia v. Blue Cross/Blue Shield, (court found treatment was not "experimental" and/or language of exclusion was ambiguous under *de novo* standard) (Motion for Summary Judgment; plaintiff prevailed; case settled)

B. Federal District Courts

Adams v. Blue Cross/Blue Shield of Md., Inc., 757 F. Supp. 661 (D. Md. 1991) ("ABMT not "experimental" for breast cancer; decision to deny coverage overturned under either de novo or 'arbitrary and capricious' standard")

Bucci v. Blue Cross-Blue Shield of Conn., Inc., 764 F. Supp. 728 (D. Conn. 1991) ("denial of coverage for ABMT for breast cancer patient arbitrary and capricious")

Dozsa v. Crum & Forster Insurance, 716 F Supp. 131 (D. N.J. 1989) (breast cancer; HDC/ABMT)

Duckwitz v. General American Life Insurance Company, 1993 WL 42186, No. 93 C 739 (N.D. Ill. Feb. 18, 1993)

Dynamic Engineering Inc. v. CHAMPUS, 850 F. Supp 459 (E.D. Vir. 1994) (Stage IV breast cancer, HDC/PSCR; unreasonable for the plan to determine that the treatment is experimental.)

Harris v. Blue Cross Blue Shield of Missouri, No. 92–CV–2427 (CEJ) (U.S. Dist. Ct. E. Mo. Dec. 18, 1992)

Kekis v. Blue Cross and Blue Shield, 815 F. Supp. 571 (N.D.N.Y. 1993)

Kulakowski v. Rochester Hosp. Serv. Corp., 779 F. Supp. 710 (W.D.N.Y. 1991) ("preliminary injunction granted in favor of breast cancer patient; decision that ABMT is 'experimental' is arbitrary and capricious")

Pirozzi v. Blue Cross-Blue Shield of Va., 741 F. Supp. 586 (E.D. Va. 1990) ("de novo standard of review applied; ABMT not 'experimental' for treatment of breast cancer" *Helman*, 803 F. Supp. 1407, 1413)

Reiff v. Blue Cross and Blue Shield of Okla., No. 90–C–1030–E (N.D. Okla, Jan. 1991)

Scalamandre v. Oxford Health Plans (NY.), Inc., et al., 1993 U.S. Dist. LEXIS 8596 (E.D.N.Y. June 15, 1993) (ERISA action court awarded $164,041.02 in coverage with prejudgment interest, plus costs, disbursements and attorney fees for HDC/ABMT for breast cancer of policyholder's now deceased wife after a 5-day trial)

Stewart v. Hewlett-Packard Co., No. 90–875–A (E.D. Va. Aug. 7, 1990)

Thomas v. Blue Cross and Blue Shield of Mass. Inc., No. 90–10831–H (D. Mass. Apr. 5, 1990)

White v. Caterpillar, Inc., 765 F. Supp. 1418 (W.D. Mo.) (injunction *affirmed* in unpublished decision reported by memorandum 965 F. 2d 564 (8th Cir. Ct. 1991); vacated pursuant to settlement No. 91–0535–CV–W–F (Nov. 24, 1992)

C. Federal Court of Appeals

Dahl-Eimers v. Mutual of Omaha Life Ins. Co., 986 F. 2d 1379 (11th Circuit. 1993) (breast cancer; HDC–ABMT; held phrase "considered experimental" in policy was ambiguous; vacated and remanded district court decision)

Farley v. Benefit Trust Life Insurance, No. 90–761C(7), (U.S. Dist. Ct. E. Mo. Oct. 17, 1991) (conclusion of law ¶¶15–17, pp18–20) (Hon. Jean M. Hamilton) affirmed 979 F. 2d 653 (8th Cir. Ct. 1992) on insurer's cross-appeal challenging finding not experimental/investigative.

Fuja, Kenneth, as Personal Representative of the Estate of Grace R. Fuja, deceased v. Benefit Trust Life Insurance Company, 18 F.3d 1405 (N.D. Ill. 1992) No. 92–C–7542 (preliminary injunction and trial on merits consolidated; held policy covered HDC/ABMT for breast cancer applying de novo standard) On appeal it was not disputed that the treatment is "required and appropriate for care of [breast cancer]", or that it is "given in accordance with generally accepted principles of medical practice in the U.S. at the time furnished" or that it was "not deemed to be experimental, educational or investigational in nature by any appropriate technological assessment body established by any state or federal government". However, it was reversed by the 7th Circuit (No. 93–1150, 1994) solely on grounds that contract exclusion for treatment provided "in connection with medical or other research" was not unambiguous and that the treatment is "still under investigation in medically recognized and accepted research studies."

Mason v. Missouri Health Insurance Pool, No. 94CC055669 (Cir. Ct. Boone County Apr. 28, 1994, Hon. Gene Hamilton)

Simmons v. Blue Cross/Blue Shield of Md., Inc., No. 3115202 (Cir. Ct. Anne Arundel County, Md. Oct 15, 1990)

Taylor v. Blue Cross/Blue Shield of Mich., No. 91–21861–CK (Cir. Ct. Marquette County, Mich. June 17, 1992), appeal pending, (Ct. App. Mich. 1992)

White v. Caterpillar, Inc., 765 F. Supp. 1418 (W.D. Mo. 1991), aff'd without published opinion, No. 91–2491WM (8th Cir. 1991) ABMT sought for breast cancer patient; court found that ABMT "investigational" exclusion "arbitrary and capricious"; temporary injunction granted")

Ms. NORTON. Who would like to speak next?

Mr. Carter.

Mr. CARTER. Good afternoon. My name is Richard Carter.

I am an attorney in Alexandria, Virginia. I have handled about 300 or so breast cancer cases in which the denial was based on experimental exclusions. In every one of those cases, based on experimental exclusion, the people got into the hospital and got covered. The result of it resulted in eight trials, all of which were successful.

I think that shows that there is a certain element of good faith lacking in the argument that these are treatments which aren't suitable for insurance coverage. And I think in the discussion today by the OPM that OPM tried to move this away from whether or not this is something that is suitable for insurance coverage and instead tried to talk about what is the state-of-the-art of medicine in its highest form.

Now, in doing so, they talked about clinical trials. And just very quickly, there are clinical trials and there are clinical trials. Every patient that I have ever represented has been on a clinical trial. I would urge you to mandate OPM to provide coverage for every person with breast cancer on an approved clinical trial. That is something they clearly don't do. It certainly gives the power of control.

You have NCI-approved protocols at the best academics institutions in America. There are 140 institutions that give this treatment around the country. I have represented people all over the country. There are all good institutions. It would keep you away from having to have Podunk hospital performing this. It would move research ahead.

More importantly, it would give us treatment. And I suggest to this committee that that is not inconsistent with how OPM and the carriers treat insurance coverage for other forms of cancer. Let's face it, the real world situation is there are 145,000 women a year that get breast cancer.

There are 28,000 people in the United States that get lymphoma every year. Lymphoma is considered and has been the subject of much testimony and trials across the country. Lymphoma is treated with high-dose chemotherapy. It has always been referred to as a home-run therapy.

And yet when you compare the objective criteria of toxicities, cure rates, long-term disease-free survival, remission, types of other complications, everything down the board, lymphoma and breast cancer are almost indistinguishable. It appears that the only difference between lymphoma and breast cancer is the fact that breast cancer seems to have a higher initial complete response rate. In other words, more people with breast cancer have their tumor disappear.

I don't think anybody can argue if you don't have any tumor, you are probably better off. Well, it is a little better with breast cancer, not worse. The difference is that nobody has ever given this a good look. They look at 145,000 people. They figure there is going to be this cost thing and they don't want to cover it. And that is the bottom line.

Now, let's look at what the insurance industry does look at. If you take the five major carriers in the United States, the big five—Aetna, Prudential, Travelers, MetLife—they all cover this, uniformly covered. In fact, in the Aetna plans that participate in the Federal employee health benefits, their HMO covers this.

Why would the big five refuse to cover things that the Federal Government or—excuse me, why would the big five pay for things when the Federal Government has to refuse? Why does medicaid pay for this? Why do state employees in Maryland have this as a mandated part of their coverage?

Why did the state assembly in Virginia go to a mandated coverage for this? Why is it that most people who have ERISA plans, if you work at Woodworth & Lothrop and you have their health plan, you get it covered? Why is it Federal workers aren't covered? Blue Cross and the OPM have suggested that these NCI trials need to work their way out.

Now, every doctor in the United States who works at an academic medical institution, I think, would agree the clinical trials are appropriate for Stage II and Stage III breast cancer, which are primary breast cancers. Everybody agrees on that. And so they haven't had much trouble accruing people for the primary—the Stage II, Stage III trials.

On the other hand, when it comes to Stage IV breast cancer, many institutions do not believe that it is ethical when you have somebody with metastatic breast cancer, who has an eight-month window before the cancer comes back, most of those institutions do not believe that it is ethical to have a clinical trial where, on one hand, you have a treatment that you know isn't going to work and, on the other hand, a treatment that does.

Georgetown University Lombardi Cancer Center is run by Dr. Mark Lippman who is the former head of breast oncology at the National Cancer Institute. This is someone that understands this.

He testified in November in 1990 in the United States District Court in Baltimore that it would be unethical to have randomized treatments when you know that one treatment here for metastatic breast cancer has a chance of working and one where you know the results are going to be dismal. Similarly, Johns Hopkins University does not participate in randomized Stage IV clinical trials, nor does Fairfax in Virginia. Those are the three biggest cancer institutions in this region. None of them will participate in randomized trials for Stage IV.

What does that mean? That means that out of the 90 or so institutions on the randomized NCI study, only 14 of them will participate in this when it looks at metastatic breast cancer. What that means is it takes much longer for the necessary number of people to accrue. If we wait for Stage III or Phase III clinical trials to decide whether to cover this treatment for breast cancer, it is going to take far too long. The evidence is here. I would suggest that we move on this right now.

Thank you.

Ms. NORTON. Thank you very much, Mr. Carter.

[The prepared statement of Mr. Carter follows:]

PREPARED STATEMENT OF RICHARD CARTER, ESQUIRE, HUDGINS, CARTER & COLEMAN

My name is Richard Carter. I am an attorney with the law firm of Hudgins Carter & Coleman in Alexandria, Virginia, and I am an Adjunct Professor of Law at Georgetown University Law Center. I would like to thank you for the opportunity to appear here today on a subject that means life or death for so many young women.

The FEHBA plan has a goal of providing competitive health benefits to federal workers to remain competitive with private enterprises. The Office of Personnel Management's policy on breast cancer makes that a lie. If a woman in Maryland, for instance, has metastatic breast cancer and works for a private employer or the state government, she is covered for the high-dose chemotherapy treatment she needs. If she doesn't work, Medicaid pays. Only the federal worker gets the death sentence. I recently helped a woman with a nine month old baby in New Orleans get on Medicaid because her federal plan would not pay for her bone marrow transplant. She is now getting treatment.

For the past four years, our law firm has handled over 300 cases involving high-dose chemotherapy with autologous bone marrow transplant (HDC/ABMT) as a treatment for aggressive cancers. At least 85% of these cases have involved coverage denials for HDC/ABMT for use with breast cancer. The carriers in those cases, like OPM, turned down high-dose chemotherapy for breast cancer because they said that "HDC/ABMT for the treatment of breast cancer is dangerous and of unproven effectiveness" and they denied coverage based on the use of the "experimental" exclusion. I have handled cases for people as far away as Arizona, California and Washington state and for people who work on Capitol Hill. Not one case initially denied as an experimental treatment has not eventually received coverage.

Sixty to eighty percent of those cases were settled without any court intervention at all. The balance of cases were filed in various United States District Courts around the country. We have only had to go to trial or to a hearing six to eight times, and in every case in which there was a trial on whether this was an experimental treatment, the patient won and the insurer was required to provide coverage.

The litigated cases have been aggressively contested by insurers who were able to hire the very finest law firms in the country. In our most recent case in United States District Court for the District of Maryland, the judge referred to the defendant's case as "contrived."

I am sure that you understand that if HDC/ABMT were really dangerous and unproven, as OPM claims, our win average would be 50% or so rather than 100%.

It is inconceivable that 275 or so carriers would voluntarily or involuntarily pay for something which was not safe and not effective. I think we can all agree that it would be difficult to fool eight federal judges when competent, effective counsel is on the other side. It is important to note that some of these cases were litigated after the patient had received the treatment and, therefore, there was little or no sympathy factor involved in the outcome.

The Memorial Sloan-Kettering Cancer Center in New York recently sued Empire Blue Cross and Blue Shield for more than $2 million, covering 21 patients receiving bone marrow transplants. In addition to patients and hospitals, the Texas Attorney General's Office sued a major insurer for consumer fraud alleging that the insurer wrongfully "misrepresented that HDC for breast cancer is experimental and/or investigational when it is not." That case was favorably resolved.

I believe that when certain insurers call this treatment "experimental," they really mean "expensive." After four years of litigating these cases, I find it impossible to believe that any of these denials are being taken for any other reason than the treatment is perceived to be expensive. Just as OPM has not been doing proper research to determine the medical value of this treatment, so, too, has it ignored medical advances which have radically reduced the cost of this treatment. When I first started doing these cases, it was not uncommon for a client to have medical bills approaching $300,000.00. If OPM and certain insurers would give this a fair and honest evaluation, they would have found out by now that the average cost has dropped tremendously; the average cost of HDC/ABMT for breast cancer at Fairfax Hospital is approximately $75,000.00 to $85,000.00, much closer to what standard therapy costs actually are.

We live in an era where there is increasing emphasis on cost effectiveness of medical treatments, and insurers like to claim that one of the reasons that they have to turn down HDC/ABMT is its effectiveness for the money. Nothing could be further from the truth.

The most recent studies of standard dose chemotherapy given to people with metastatic breast cancer show the following: Young women with breast cancer will be in remission a median of eight months. They will have a medial survival of 1.6 years with standard therapy. In fact, as numerous studies by Dr. Craig Henderson and others make clear, standard dose therapy has not been shown to increase survival of young women with aggressive breast cancer over no treatment at all.

The HDC/ABMT treatment has been used with great success at centers throughout the United States and is widely accepted as the best available care for relatively young, healthy patients with advanced breast cancer. Dr. William Peters of the Duke University Medical Center is an internationally recognized oncologist with years of experience in the successful use of this treatment. As of the end of 1992 over 600 women with breast cancer have received this treatment at Duke alone. I urge you to consider the graph he has prepared which is attached as an exhibit to this testimony. The graph shows the results of four series of patients who were followed after receiving HDC/ABMT. All of the later series show a definite "tail" or plateau in which a substantial number of people remain alive and *disease free* for as long as seven years. Since women with metastatic disease treated with conventional therapy have only a median survival of 1.6 years, this graph speaks volumes about the efficacy of this treatment. The graph plainly shows that women with metastatic disease are still alive and cancer free five and one half years after the median survivorship without HDCT. Please remember that those "survivors" who don't get HDCT frequently are very sick and have a poor quality of life.

Young women with earlier but still aggressive cancers benefit from HDCT as well. Approximately 55 to 87% of Stage II/III patients treated with conventional therapy will relapse within five years, yet the women treated with HDC/ABMT are 80% disease free at three years. At four years, 72% are still disease free, compared to only 30 to 38% of those treated with low dose therapy.

If we are concerning ourselves with bang for the buck, why are we promoting a technology of standard dose chemotherapy which has been proven to be no more effective than giving a woman an apple a day? In other words, we will spend a lot of money for something that we know won't cure you, but we are not willing to spend a little more for something that has as much as an 80% chance of providing long-term, disease-free survival.

OPM and some insurers contend that HDC/ABMT is experimental. Some Federal plans participate in the funding of randomized clinical trials to support their position that these treatments are "experimental." What they fail to tell you is that most women with breast cancer don't fit the criteria for these trials. They also fail to admit that most good cancer centers such as John Hopkins, Georgetown, and Fairfax Hospital refuse to participate in randomized trials for HDC/ABMT in breast cancer because the doctors believe HDC/ABMT is so far superior to standard treatment that randomization is unethical. They also don't tell you that they use the existence of these trials as an excuse not to pay for treatment.

Courts agree that the term "experimental" is ambiguous. Faced with such rulings, insurers have begun defining experimental exclusions which are even more devious. The following exclusion is a masterpiece of the genre:

The Medical Director of BCBSM shall have authority to determine all questions in connection with whether the use of any treatment, procedure, facility, equipment, drug, device, or supply (each of which is hereafter called a "Service") is experimental or investigative.

a. If, in making that determination, the Medical Director finds that the Service, for which a claim for benefits is made, is either:

(1) the subject of a written investigational or research protocol used by the treating facility or of another facility studying substantially the same Service; or

(2) the subject of a written informed consent used by the treating facility which refers to the Service as experimental, investigative, or research; or

(3) the subject of an on-going phase I, II, or III clinical trial, the Service shall be deemed to be experimental or investigative.

When this section is applied by Blue Cross, virtually any treatment given at major cancer centers is excluded. The above exclusion is so broad that it is meaningless; yet people are denied coverage based on it. This exclusion also points out the reasons behind some third party payors' support of the clinical trials: so long as clinical trials are conducted, companies with similar experimental exclusions need not pay.

Not every women who gets breast cancer needs HDC/ABMT; yet the people who need it have only certain death as an option. There are strict guidelines used by medical facilities to determine who are appropriate candidates. This will not open the floodgates and bankrupt FEHBA. However, one out of eight or nine women get breast cancer. This year Dr. Roy Beveridge, Director of the Bone Marrow Transplant Department of Fairfax Hospital, has had as many as 15 young women who needed the treatment but who couldn't get covered because they were federal employees.

Recently, some states such as Florida, New Hampshire, and Virginia have looked at the advisability of mandating coverage. I had the privilege of working on a task force which was successful this year in encouraging the Virginia Assembly to require all insurers doing business in Virginia to at least offer coverage for high-dose chemotherapy for breast cancer in all group policies in the state. I encourage you to do the same for federal workers.

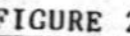

Duke University Bone Marrow Transplant Program
Time to Progression After Treatment for Breast Cancer
Probability of Continued Response
1.0
0.8
0.6
0.4
0.2
0.0
Stage IV, Prior chemo   (J Clin Oncol 11:1592 (1986)
Stage IV, No prior chemo, Proc ASCO 9:31, (1990)
CPA/cDDP/BCNU alone J. Clin Oncol 6:1368 (1988)
Stage IV, No prior chemo,
AFM → CPA/cDDP/BCNU Proc ASCO 9:30 (1990)
Stage II; 10+ LN
CAF → CPA/cDDP/BCNU Proc ASCO 9:80 (1990)
Current Programs
1985-6
1984
0 1 2 3 4 5 6 7
Years
4/90

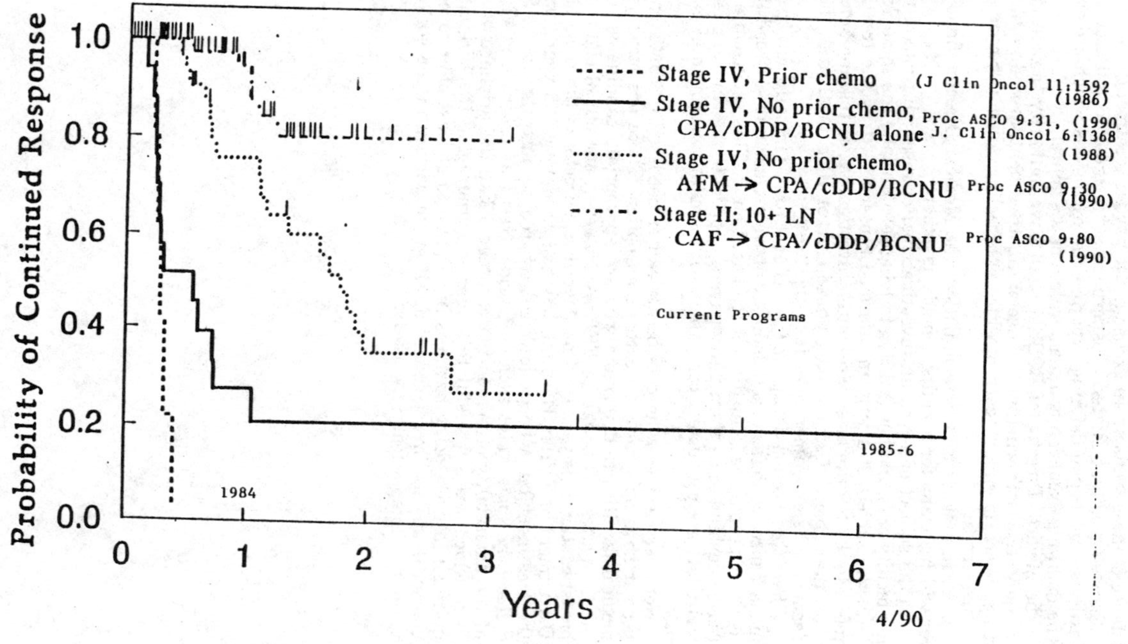

Ms. NORTON. Ms. Calder.

Ms. CALDER. Thank you, Madam Chairwoman. My name is Kimberly Calder. I am the Director of Public Policy at Cancer Care and it is an honor to represent Cancer Care before you and the members of the subcommittee.

I would like for the record to disclose I am a recent appointee to the board of directors of Empire Blue Cross/Blue Shield. I am not in any way representing Empire's position here today and, in fact, you will see the ethicacy of my organization is in conflict with the reimbursement policy of that company.

Cancer Care is a nonprofit non-meritorious sectarian social work agency established 50 years ago to help patients and their families cope with the consequences of cancer. This broad mission is carried out through the provision of comprehensive services, including professional counseling for patients, family members and the bereaved; financial assistance; information and referral; educational programs for health professionals and the public; as well as entitlement and insurance counseling.

Significantly, Cancer Care services are provided at no cost to the children or the family and the agency is supported entirely through private donations, grants, and contributions.

While Cancer Care has concentrated its program regionally through offices in New York, New Jersey, Connecticut and Long Island, its scope extends nationally as clients' needs are translated into public policy, social research, and educational programs nationwide. Full implementation of toll-free counseling services to cancer patients and families will result in the realization of the agency's eventual goal of being a direct service provider to individuals in all 50 states.

Cancer Care takes no position on access to or reimbursement for HDC with ABMT specifically. Rather, our relevant position is based squarely on our firm belief that people with cancer should have access to state-of-the-art anti-cancer therapy as recommended by cancer specialists and that they have the right to expect their insured to provide for such coverage.

As such, our position regarding coverage of an investigational therapy which is attached in my written record, provides strong support for coverage of patient care cost associated with approved clinical trials. Therefore, Cancer Care supports coverage of HDC with ABMT within the context of an approved clinical trials and whether other criteria are met, including informed consent, an approval by an institutional review board.

Notably, this position is consistent with the American Society of Clinical Oncology, the American Cancer Society, the Nation Coalition for Cancer Society, the Association of Community Cancer Centers, and other leaders in the oncology field.

Ms. CALDER. It is the position advocated by all of these groups in their statements on health care reform.

We are pleased to note that most of the major health care reform plans introduced over the last years have also incorporated the standard we support by including coverage for approved clinical trials in all their plans. It is disturbing to note, however, that none of those plans would provide for coverage for medicare recipients. Given that roughly 50 percent of all people with cancer in the Unit-

Ms. NORTON. Ms. Calder.

Ms. CALDER. Thank you, Madam Chairwoman. My name is Kimberly Calder. I am the Director of Public Policy at Cancer Care and it is an honor to represent Cancer Care before you and the members of the subcommittee.

I would like for the record to disclose I am a recent appointee to the board of directors of Empire Blue Cross/Blue Shield. I am not in any way representing Empire's position here today and, in fact, you will see the ethicacy of my organization is in conflict with the reimbursement policy of that company.

Cancer Care is a nonprofit non-meritorious sectarian social work agency established 50 years ago to help patients and their families cope with the consequences of cancer. This broad mission is carried out through the provision of comprehensive services, including professional counseling for patients, family members and the bereaved; financial assistance; information and referral; educational programs for health professionals and the public; as well as entitlement and insurance counseling.

Significantly, Cancer Care services are provided at no cost to the children or the family and the agency is supported entirely through private donations, grants, and contributions.

While Cancer Care has concentrated its program regionally through offices in New York, New Jersey, Connecticut and Long Island, its scope extends nationally as clients' needs are translated into public policy, social research, and educational programs nationwide. Full implementation of toll-free counseling services to cancer patients and families will result in the realization of the agency's eventual goal of being a direct service provider to individuals in all 50 states.

Cancer Care takes no position on access to or reimbursement for HDC with ABMT specifically. Rather, our relevant position is based squarely on our firm belief that people with cancer should have access to state-of-the-art anti-cancer therapy as recommended by cancer specialists and that they have the right to expect their insured to provide for such coverage.

As such, our position regarding coverage of an investigational therapy which is attached in my written record, provides strong support for coverage of patient care cost associated with approved clinical trials. Therefore, Cancer Care supports coverage of HDC with ABMT within the context of an approved clinical trials and whether other criteria are met, including informed consent, an approval by an institutional review board.

Notably, this position is consistent with the American Society of Clinical Oncology, the American Cancer Society, the Nation Coalition for Cancer Society, the Association of Community Cancer Centers, and other leaders in the oncology field.

Ms. CALDER. It is the position advocated by all of these groups in their statements on health care reform.

We are pleased to note that most of the major health care reform plans introduced over the last years have also incorporated the standard we support by including coverage for approved clinical trials in all their plans. It is disturbing to note, however, that none of those plans would provide for coverage for medicare recipients. Given that roughly 50 percent of all people with cancer in the Unit-

Patients turned down by their insurers for bone marrow transplant therapy who want help organizing bake sales, car washes, and door-to-door fundraising campaigns in hopes of raising $80–$100,000;

Patients who report unreasonable problems with all insurance claims subsequent to submission of a claim for a bone marrow harvest;

Patients referred for HDC with ABMT who need assistance choosing the right facility;

Patients whose HDC with ABMT therapy will be far from home who need help planning for child care while they are in treatment, including help telling their children where they're going;

Patients turned down by their insurers for such treatment who need referral to an attorney knowledgeable in this area; and

Patients who die while awaiting legal action forcing third party payers to assume fiscal responsibility before the treatment can begin.

As you know, high dose chemo followed by a bone marrow transplant or "rescue" is aggressive therapy which both patients and their families must approach as informed consumers. Cancer Care is well equipped to support those informational and decision-making needs through its counseling and educational services. Unfortunately, we are less able to help those clients who turn to us when a transplant has been recommended but denied due to the restrictive policy of the patient's insurer. The consequences of denials are financially and emotionally devastating to patients and their families. Very few families have the information, time or will necessary to battle their insurer as well as the disease itself. A very small minority of patients are willing or able to pursue legal action—often the final recourse for people fighting for their lives.

EXPERIMENTAL EXCLUSION [1]

While women with breast cancer denied access to bone marrow transplants are common in our caseload, so are patients with *other* types of cancer denied access by insurers for the same rationale—because the recommended therapy is considered "experimental" and therefore outside the scope of the insurance contract. Cancer Care has responded to this problem on behalf of all our clients by addressing changes in law and reimbursement policy that focus on the exclusion of all therapies deemed "experimental".

As you know, there is a clause common to almost every health insurance policy in the country today, referred to as the experimental exclusion, which allows insurers to deny coverage for any and all therapies deemed by them as "experimental". As documented by Drs. Peters and Rogers of the Duke University Bone Marrow Transplant Program, the pre-determinations of requests to insurers for bone marrow transplants are often "arbitrary and capricious (and are) a barrier to obtaining treatment." (New England Journal of Medicine 1994: 330:473–7).

The original purpose of the experimental exclusion was reasonable and based on the insurers' responsibility to the insured individual, as well as to all insureds paying premiums, to prevent the underwriting of treatments with no medical justification, otherwise known as "quackery". In recent years, however, the experimental exclusion has become the means by which third party payers have avoided paying for a wide range of medically indicated, necessary and high quality treatments.

The experimental exclusion, and the entire question of standard vs. experimental treatment, has been the subject of controversy and debate whose scope far exceeds this Subcommittee's immediate concern. Nonetheless, the Subcommittee should be aware that this subject consistently dominates policy discussions within the cancer community. In fact, there is arguably no more critical issue for this community (including clinicians, researchers and patient groups alike) in the health care reform debate, than the question of coverage of investigational therapy.

CANCER CARE POLICY

Cancer Care takes no position on access to, or reimbursement for, HDC with ABMT specifically. Rather, our relevant position is based squarely in our firm belief that people with cancer should have access to state-of-the-art anti-cancer therapy as recommended by cancer specialists, and that they have the right to expect their insurer to provide for such coverage.

---

[1] Note that the term "experimental" is commonly used by insurers, while "investigational" is the term of choice among physicians and researchers. Both refer to therapies, including drugs and procedures, whose safety and efficacy is either under evaluation, or not specifically approved for marketing by the Food & Drug Administration. "Crossover therapy" is a new term for the same, as coined by S.J. Reiser in his recent article. Health Affairs, Summer, 1994)

As such, our position regarding coverage of investigational therapy, as attached, provides strong support for coverage of patient care costs associated with approved clinical trials. Therefore, Cancer Care supports coverage of HDC with ABMT *when provided within the context of an approved clinical trial,* and when other criteria for clinical trials are met, including informed consent, and approval by an institutional review board. Notably, this position is consistent with positions of the American Society of Clinical Oncology, American Cancer Society, National Coalition for Cancer Survivorship, Candlelighters' Childhood Cancer Foundation, Association of Community Cancer Centers, and other leaders in oncology. It is the position advocated by all of these groups in their statements on health care reform.

THE IMPORTANCE OF STANDARDS

In the case of investigational therapy, insurance companies generally assume there is no demonstration of safety and effectiveness, which is the usual standard for insurance coverage. However, in the case of serious or life-threatening conditions, the Food and Drug Administration (FDA) and others have recognized that a more flexible standard is required in order to provide patients with such diseases with the best available care. In place of the usual safety and effectiveness requirement, the cancer community as well as AIDS groups advocate a different standard under which patients should be covered for treatment provided pursuant to peer reviewed, high quality clinical trials.

This position taken by Cancer Care and other groups uses clear and concise standards concerning the requirements for an "approved" clinical trial. Clearly, this standard excludes coverage for some HDC with ABMT treatments, and we have been criticized for taking this more restrictive approach. Yet, authorization of coverage of treatments meeting no unified and objective standard would be irresponsible, even in the face of life-threatening illness.

Further, it is critically important that standards used in assessment of investigational therapies be impartial, and uniformly applied to all insureds. The Blue Cross Blue Shield Association, for example, has devised its own Technology Assessment Program, as well as its own five point criteria for use by member Blues organizations in their own determination of coverage for investigational therapy. These criteria are commonly criticized by attorneys and others knowledgeable of these issues as being entirely too vague and self-interested to be credible.

Within this difficult debate, it is important to assure to the patient, the family and their insurer, that the highest standards of care will not be abandoned. We believe our position supports access to the highest standards of care, and that people with cancer have the greatest likelihood of a beneficial outcome because of it.

HEALTH CARE REFORM LEGISLATION AND COVERAGE OF INVESTIGATIONAL THERAPIES

We are pleased to note that most of the major health care reform plans introduced over the last year have also incorporated the standard we support by including coverage for approved by clinical trials. Under these plans, insurance policies would have to cover patient care costs in peer-reviewed trials, including those approved by the FDA, the National Institutes of Health, the Department of Defense, and the Department of Veterans Affairs. We believe this approach will provide payment for most of the high quality clinical research.

While the exact scope of the House Majority bill's benefits package is not yet known, similar coverage has been included in legislation drafted by the Administration, all four of the major congressional committees that voted on health care reform (the House Ways & Means, House Education and Labor, Senate Finance and Senate Labor and Human Resources Committees), and the Senate Majority. Therefore it appears very likely that through health care reform the standard supported by the cancer community and others will become the new standard required to be adopted by the insurance industry.

It is disturbing to note, however, that none of the plans would provide for such coverage for Medicare recipients. Given that roughly 50% of all people with cancer in the U.S. are 65 years of age or older, it is profoundly short sighted, unfair, and antithetical to the goal of universal, comprehensive coverage to allow for different benefit packages for people with cancer simply as a consequence of age. The individuals of this Subcommittee could make a major contribution to the legislation and people with cancer by sponsoring an amendment to extend this provision to Medicare recipients.

CONCLUSION AND RECOMMENDATION

The question you and I have been asked to address today is limited to whether or not the Federal Employee Health Benefit Program (FEHBP) should now include coverage for high dose chemotherapy with autologous bone marrow transplant for women with breast cancer. I respectfully submit to you that this is too narrow a question. Rather, I encourage the Subcommittee to address the current and future need of all Program participants, not just breast cancer patients, to state-of-the-art anti-cancer treatments. Providing FEHBP coverage for patient care costs in approved clinical trials would acknowledge the very dynamic nature of cancer treatment, and would, once and for all, settle these issues without requiring constant re-examination of the benefit package and available data on safety and efficacy. Further, it would provide for a reimbursement policy supporting access to high quality care, as well as continued medical progress through clinical research. Finally, adoption of this standard would guarantee that coverage decisions are based on appropriate and objective authority acting in the best interests of patient care and scientific advancement.

Thank you for this opportunity to comment.

POLICY STATEMENT ON THIRD PARTY PAYER COVERAGE OF INVESTIGATIONAL TREATMENT

Cancer patients assume their physicians recommend certain treatments for them because they have the best likelihood for success, and they assume their insurance will cover treatments recommended by qualified physicians. However, in the treatment of cancer, therapies with "the best likelihood for success" are often still under investigation and not yet approved by the Food & Drug Administration. Access to those treatments is therefore only available through participation in clinical trials.

Increasingly, however, patients' ability to participate in clinical trials is limited by reimbursement policies of third-party payers. Typically, the actual drug under investigation is provided to the patient at no cost. The ancillary costs, including hospitalization, physician fees, lab fees and supplies are billed to the patient, just as they would be for standard treatment. The patient in turn seeks reimbursement from his/her insurer, which historically honored those claims as legitimate costs eligible for reimbursement.

In recent years, an increasing number of third-party payers have denied coverage for costs associated with participation in clinical trials. These insurers claim that the treatment is experimental, and therefore outside the scope of the insurance contract. The "experimental exclusion" has no standard definition and is therefore applied in a seemingly random fashion by commercial carriers, HMOs, Medicare carriers and state controlled Medicaid programs.[1]

The consequences of these practices are financially and emotionally devastating to patients and their families. Very few families have the information, time or will necessary to battle their insurer as well as the disease itself. A very small minority of patients are willing or able to pursue legal action—often the final recourse for people fighting for their lives. The toll of this problem on physicians' treatment choices and time are well-documented.[2]

There are many sound arguments offered by both sides of this often complex and controversial debate. However, the essential needs of cancer patients are simple and unchanging. As with all manner of health care services, patients must be assured access to medically-indicated state-of-the-art treatment.

When a patient chooses a course of treatment involving a clinical trial, that treatment should be covered by the insurer provided informed consent requirements are satisfied and basic standards of safety and efficacy are assured. Reimbursement for new therapies still under investigation should not be denied when the following circumstances are present:

(a) Treatment is being provided pursuant to a clinical trial which has been approved by the National Institutes of Health (NIH) in cooperation with the National Cancer Institute (NCI), any of its cancer centers, cooperative groups or community clinical oncology programs; the Food and Drug Administration in the form of an Investigational New Drug (IND) exemption; the Department of Veteran Affairs; or a qualified nongovernmental research entity as identified in the guidelines for NCI cancer center support grants; and

(b) The proposed therapy has been reviewed and approved by a qualified institutional review board (IRB); and

(c) The facility and personnel providing the treatment are capable of doing so by virtue of their experience or training; and

---

[1] Lee N. Newcomer, Md, MS. "Defining Experimental Therapy—A Third-Party Payer's Dilemma", The New England Journal of Medicine, Vol. 323:24, December 13, 1990, pp. 1702–4.

[2] *Reimbursement Policies for Off-Label Drugs,* U.S. General Accounting Office/PEMD–01–14, September 1991.

138

(d) The patients receiving the investigational treatment meet all protocol or compassionate use requirements; and

(e) There is no clearly superior, non-investigational alternative to the protocol treatment; and

(f) The available clinical or preclinical data provide a reasonable expectation that the protocol treatment will be at least as efficacious as the alternative.

In addition, institutions and clinicians providing these treatments must demonstrate willingness and ability to work with patients to resolve their party payer disputes to assure access to the therapies they recommend. At a minimum, patients must be informed that insurance coverage may be problematic as soon as a clinical trial is recommended. Institutions and physicians must provide scientific evidence of efficacy and other supportive documentation to the patient, the patient's agent or the insurer, in a prompt and professional manner. Physicians should never fail to recommend their first choice of therapy to the patient for fear of an insurance denial of coverage.

Ms. NORTON. Thank you very much.

Let me begin by asking Ms. Groch, your testimony seems to imply that there is collusion between OPM and companies who have now moved from giving as a reason for denying coverage here that the treatment is investigative to simply taking it out of the contract, and that OPM is facilitating this process?

Ms. GROCH. I do not have any doubt that that is the situation. This is not a coincidental thing. These are contracts obviously that are negotiated between the parties. And if OPM, in fact, believed that the treatment was—if the issue to OPM was whether or not the treatment is effective or at least as effective as standard chemotherapy as they have presented the issue here, then they would have had no need to change the contracts to put in an exclusionary clause. The only reason to put that in was to assist the insurance companies in winning their cases in court.

Ms. NORTON. Do you know of OPM having done this before in any other instances?

Ms. GROCH. I know that in every case that I have litigated involving the FEHBA, OPM has submitted affidavits in support of the insurance companies.

Ms. NORTON. In cases with facts radically different from the facts before us?

Ms. GROCH. No, in the ABMT cases.

Ms. NORTON. I am trying to see if this is normal practice for OPM or whether they have started to do that with this particular treatment?

Ms. GROCH. I don't have the answer to that question, perhaps Mr. Carter has.

Mr. CARTER. Madam Chairman, I had a case in Federal district court in Baltimore, and every case that I have ever read involving OPM or its predecessor and health benefits involved efforts by OPM to get out of the case, to emphasize that they were not a proper party. In fact, that is what the regulations indicate. I had a case in Maryland on the other hand, where the OPM intervened so that not only did I have three lawyers from the insurance company trying to kill my client, but two from OPM.

Ms. NORTON. With respect to this treatment?

Mr. CARTER. They intervened in the court case.

Ms. NORTON. On the side of the insurer?

Mr. CARTER. Yes.

Ms. GROCH. I had the same insurance in Philips versus Blue Cross in Colorado Federal Court of Appeals. I won that case on a jurisdictional issue, and Blue Cross appealed. And the Department of Justice filed an amicus brief on behalf of the insurance company against the Federal employee.

Mr. CARTER. Mine was at the trial court level.

Ms. GROCH. By the way, the Tenth Circuit didn't agree with Blue Cross or the Department of Justice and has just ruled in favor of the plaintiff and said there is no Federal jurisdiction.

Ms. NORTON. One of the things that the subcommittee simply has to find out is whether or not OPM is assuming a different role from its historic role and the role that Federal employees believe it is assuming? Staying out of it is one thing. Getting in it on the side of the insurer against the employee seems to me to call upon them for an explanation which we have not yet received and indeed as Mr. Myers said, I thought they indicated the opposite.

Mr. MYERS. I am going back through the testimony now.

Mr. CARTER. They are quick to emphasize that they don't really have anything to do with coverage determinations, yet, you have to appeal to them. And on one hand, they say they don't make individual determinations and that is in the regulations, and in fact they said that today, I think it was my understanding, but yet at the same time, they will say that because this was a decision of an administrative agency, that it is only subject to arbitrary and capricious review.

Ms. NORTON. I was discussing with staff this appeal in light of OPM's assertion that of course we don't have anything to do with deciding what to cover or not to cover. And it seems to me that as perhaps as costs have gone up and as lines have been blurred generally between doctors and insurers and between providers and others, that OPM's role may now be confused and the subcommittee has to look at that role so that at least employees understand whose side who is on.

At the very least, they deserve notice of that. If they want a role, that is in greater partnership with the insurer, they ought to justify that role. Everybody ought to know it. And they ought to explain it to this committee so it can be approved.

And in appealing, I don't know that insurance companies appeal to this. If employees are appealing to them for some kind of neutral here, the question becomes how they perceive that neutrality and whether they are playing the role of a genuine neutral?

Ms. GROCH. What happens in these cases is that the employee gets a denial from the insurance company and then even if they do not exercise their right to review by OPM, the insurance company appeals to OPM. And the insurance company then gets its rubber stamp from OPM. It usually takes about 24 hours for OPM to do its, quote, review of the Blue Cross or Mail Handlers' denial. They do not look at the medical evidence in the record because that is not the issue before them. They simply write a letter and say the contract excludes it, therefore, we back the insurance company. And then they always have this line that says, we regret the difficult situation your medical condition puts you in, et cetera. And then OPM does something else. They say, but we have these clinical randomized trials. And what is happening there by saying "we have the clinical randomized trials", on the one hand, and on the other hand you can't get insurance reimbursement because we are going to back the insurance company in denying you, OPM is funneling patients into the NCI study by a coercive measure. I don't think there is any question.

If on the one hand you are told you can only get in treatment if you go into the NCI study, the randomized NCI study, then of course it is coercive. And OPM, as I guess a sister agency with NCI, recognizing that NCI has been having difficulty getting its patient population to finish the study that the scientists want to finish, is cooperating with the insurance companies, on the one hand, and NCI, on the other hand, to deny them the coverage and the insurance and funnel those patients into the study. The result being, if you have money, you have choice; if you have no money, you have no choice.

Ms. NORTON. There is a vote on, and I am going to have Mr. Myers ask the remainder of questions because I don't think we can come back after this one.

Mr. Myers, do you have any questions?

Mr. MYERS. I only have a couple of questions. I have concerns about this intervention by OPM. It really underlies everything we have been talking about today. And even though I went back through and I don't think specifically—I wish we had talked to you sooner, asked them that question but it is certainly implied throughout their statement. Of course, you were all here when the one gentleman testified.

It says the insurer, not OPM, determined the application of these general exclusions. OPM doesn't have the expertise nor would it be appropriate to make independent determination as to reasonableness, medical necessity or efficacy of medical procedure. It certainly implies here they don't do those kinds of things. And this is the whole thing we are concerned about. Do our Federal employees have less access to medical——

Mr. CARTER. Your Federal employees have no rights. That is absolutely correct. Your Federal employees have absolutely no rights when it comes to breast cancer. They are stuck. Now if they have stage II or stage III breast cancer and they have to go into a randomized study, that is not that big a deal because it if doesn't work then they can get, perhaps, high dose chemotherapy down the road.

But where it is a death sentence is for people with metastatic breast cancer. Metastatic breast cancer is going to kill them. There is just no other way around it. The only choice they have is getting high dose chemotherapy, at which point they have a 20 to 30 percent chance of long-term disease-free survival. There are people out nine years, 10 years that are alive with no tumors that should have been dead eight-and-a-half years ago. Those people don't have any rights at all. One, they won't qualify to fit into the randomized trial anyway, and secondly, they really don't have any access to effective judicial intervention.

Mr. MYERS. That concerns all of us and that is what this hearing is all about, making sure that our employees are not treated differently.

One other thing. In your testimony you quoted Dr. Marc Lippman—the Federal court in Baltimore. At the same time that you say that was the best, the only treatment—he was my wife's doctor and he gave her just regular chemo.

Mr. CARTER. High dose chemotherapy is only used for certain subsets of patients. Your wife was lucky, she didn't need it.

Mr. MYERS. She was stage IV, very advanced stage IV, with metastasized. I am going after Marc. Here he testified in Baltimore and you got him in trouble with me.

We are very concerned about this and we thank you for your testimony. I hope that your job will be made a little easier. Of course we may be taking clients away from you in the future.

Mr. CARTER. Please put us out of business.

Ms. GROCH. That is exactly what we want.

Mr. MYERS. The lives of these people are very much more important than the legal profession, or the medical profession.

Ms. GROCH. I would like, if I may, make one last point and that is that Mr. Smith in his opening statement said we are willing to change the coverage provisions even in mid-year. We know that, of course, the open window is November for people to select their policies for next year and those policies are in all probability written and contracts signed but he has said they are willing to change them midyear and we should not have another 15 months of women dying because they are not getting coverage who are Federal employees.

Thank you.

Ms. NORTON. Thank you very much.

First of all, I want to thank my colleague, Mr. Myers, for bringing so much real life experience to his questions. I found it a very important aspect at this hearing. That is exactly what we need to know. What we are talking about is not an abstraction here and you kept us understanding that throughout your very good questions. I want to thank the three of you very much, because this is a hearing that has gone on longer than most but, if I may say so, it has been more important than most. And your testimony has been indispensable.

If it had not been included in the record, I can see now by what you said, the record would have been very incomplete. And I want to thank each of you for staying through a very long day to help us to make a complete record with very vital testimony.

Ms. GROCH. Thank you. If there is anything that we have that might supplement the record, may we submit it?

Ms. NORTON. Yes, the record will be open for 30 days for your submissions.

Mr. MYERS. If we can save one life, all of our time has been worth it and I think there is the possibility of saving many.

Ms. NORTON. As I said before, the fact that OPM, so far as I can see, for the first time today has said it will consider even midyear allowing reimbursement or requiring reimbursement for all forms of trials, and not the narrow form alone that reimbursement is allowed for. If that in fact is the case, I believe that the hearing has moved us some considerable distance.

Ms. GROCH. Thanks to your effective cross-examination.

Ms. NORTON. Thank you very much.

Mr. MYERS. Thank you.

Ms. NORTON. The hearing is adjourned.

[Whereupon, at 3:06 p.m., the subcommittee was adjourned.]

[Additional material submitted for the record follows:]

Hon. ELEANOR HOLMES NORTON
Chairwoman, Subcommittee On Compensation and Employee Benefits, Washington, DC.

DEAR MADAM CHAIRMWOMAN: Enclosed is written testimony submitted by my constituents Kenneth and Connie Justis for the August 11 Subcommittee on Compensation and Employee Benefits hearing on the Federal Employees Health Benefit Plan (FEHBP) and breast cancer treatments.

Kenneth Justis is employed by the National Oceanic and Atmospheric Administration in Wallops, Virginia. He has insurance with the Government Employees Hospital Association (GEHA) under FEHBP. His wife, Connie, was first diagnosed with breast cancer over nine years ago. Due to the responsibilities of caring for Connie, transporting her to and from treatment and doctor visits and working 12-hour shifts each day, Kenneth was unable to travel to Washington to testify in person. I am pleased to bring to your attention written testimony regarding high dose chemotherapy and autologous bone marrow transplant (HDC/ABMT) as treatment for breast cancer.

I would appreciate your including the enclosed testimony in the proceedings from the August 11 hearing in this matter. I believe this situation is one which merits a great deal of attention and hope that the testimony of my constituents will prove helpful in the Subcommittee's investigative process.

With kind regards, I am
    Sincerely yours,

HERBERT H. BATEMAN,
Member of Congress.

PREPARED STATEMENT OF KENNETH AND CONNIE JUSTIS

My name is Kenneth Justis and I work for the National Oceanic and Atmospheric Administration Wallops CDA station in Virginia. I have insurance coverage with the Government Employees Hospital Association (GEHA) under the Federal Employees Health Benefit Plan (FEHBP). My wife, Connie, has battled recurring breast cancer for almost a decade. I am submitting written testimony in lieu of appearing in person because I am unable to travel to Washington. Because Connie and I live some distance from any neighbors or hospital, I must care for her at home and we spend approximately six hours each day travelling to and from doctors' offices and hospitals. In addition, I work shifts of 12 hours each day. If it had been at all possible, we certainly would have made the trip to Washington to testify, and if Connie recovers and there are hearings in the future, we would be pleased to participate.

In 1985, Connie was first diagnosed with breast cancer, at which time she underwent chemotherapy and radiation. Since that time, she has visited her doctors regularly.

In March of 1994, Connie experienced difficulty when walking and had pain in her side for more than a week. She had four days of tests at Virginia Beach General Hospital (VBGH) and an office visit with Dr. Michael Steinberg of Hematology-Oncology of Tidewater. The tests showed that the cancer had spread to her ovaries, stomach and liver. Consequently, she underwent a hysterectomy, performed by Dr. George Kemp of Gynecologists of Tidewater. Two weeks later, she began chemotherapy at VBGH, consisting of a series of inpatient procedures along with home health care injections and outpatient treatments. The chemotherapy caused Connie to have badly swollen and blistered hands and feet, as well as nausea. In addition, she has been advised by doctors to maintain only minimal contact with anyone outside of the family because of the possibility of infection.

When Connie began chemotherapy in April, we also were informed by Dr. Steinberg that she would need to undergo a bone marrow transplant. At that time, I called GEHA to ask if the bone marrow procedure would be covered. I was informed verbally by GEHA and by her doctors that the procedure would be covered.

In July, Connie began the high dose chemotherapy and autologous bone marrow transplant (HDC/ABMT) program through Response Technologies. During the first treatment, we were told that GEHA had denied coverage. I have attached a copy of the letter from GEHA dated July 6, 1994. It states that GEHA does not cover HDC/ABMT for treatment of breast cancer. The letter also informs us of a clinical research trial sponsored by the National Cancer Institute, which involves the use of HDC/ABMT as treatment for breast cancer. Unfortunately, Connie already had begun her treatment and was not eligible. She had begun the treatment after being informed by doctors that it was vitally important and she could not wait.

As you may know, on October 29, 1993, many Members of Congress sent a letter to James King, Director of the Office of Personnel Management (OPM), requesting that OPM require FEHBP insurance carries to cover HDC/ABMT for breast cancer. The response stated that it will take time to establish data proving that the treatment is effective enough to outweigh the risks. I have attached copies of the letter to Mr. King and his response.

Connie and I understand that there are risks involved in the HDC/ABMT treatment, but we have decided, as anyone would, that we will take the risks if the treatment can save Connie's life. It is not the procedure itself that is a problem, because it is covered for leukemia, Hodgkin's testicular and ovarian cancers. Presently, the legal counsel for Response Technologies is in the process of attempting to obtain payment from GEHA for Connie and others they are treating.

I share with you this information in hopes that FEHBP will give serious consideration to covering high dose chemotherapy and autologous bone marrow transplant (HDC/ABMT) as treatment for breast cancer. Connie and I appreciate the opportunity to tell our story and hope this testimony is helpful.

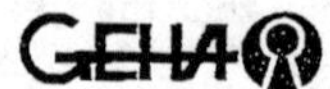

GOVERNMENT EMPLOYEES HOSPITAL ASSOCIATION, INC.
P.O. BOX 10304 / KANSAS CITY, MISSOURI 64171-0304 / 816-753-1260
(CLAIM INQUIRIES – 816-257-5500)

July 6, 1994

E. Paul Getaz, MD   COPY
6005 Park Ave Ste 130-B
Memphis TN 38119-5206

Re: Connie Justis - Patient
     Kenneth A. Justis – Member
     ID# 225-56-6670

Dear Dr. Getaz:

This will acknowledge receipt of the preauthorization request for high
dose chemotherapy supported by autologous bone marrow transplant or
peripheral blood stem cell reinfusion for the diagnosis of breast
cancer.

Page 19 of the 1994 GEHA Brochure describes coverage for transplants.
GEHA Members are provided with the Brochure when they join the Plan.
We quote the applicable provisions:

> "The following human organ/tissue transplant
> procedures are covered, subject to the
> conditions and limitations below, and only when
> the recipient is covered by this Plan:
>
> . Allogenic bone marrow transplants, limited to
>   patients with (1) Acute leukemia, (2)
>   Advanced Hodgkin's lymphoma, (3) Advanced
>   non-Hodgkin's lymphoma, (4) Advanced
>   Neuroblastoma (limited to children over age
>   one), (5) Aplastic anemia, (6) Chronic
>   myelogenous leukemia, (7) Infantile malignant
>   osteoporosis, (8) Severe combined
>   immunodeficiency, (9) Thalassemia major, or
>   (10) Wiskott-Aldrich syndrome.
>
> . Autologous bone marrow transplants
>   (autologous stem cell support) and autologous
>   peripheral stem cell support, limited to
>   patients with (1) Acute lymphocytic, or
>   non-lymphocytic leukemia, (2) Advanced
>   Hodgkin's lymphoma, (3) Advanced
>   non-Hodgkin's lymphoma, (4) Advanced
>   neuroblastoma (limited to children over age
>   one), or (5) Testicular, Mediastinal,
>   Retroperitoneal and Ovarian germ cell
>   tumors;

(2)

. Cornea, heart, heart/lung, kidney and liver
transplants;

. Pancreas transplants, limited to patients
whose condition is not treatable by insulin
therapy;

. Single or double lung transplants, limited to
patients for the following end-stage
pulmonary diseases (1) Primary fibrosis, (2)
pulmonary hypertention, or (3) Emphysema;
double lung transplants, limited to patients
with cystic fibrosis..."

and

"What Is not Covered - Services or supplies for
or related to surgical transplant procedures
for artificial or human organ/tissue
transplants not listed as specifically covered
such as breast cancer. Related services or
supplies include administration of high dose
chemotherapy when supported by transplant
procedures."

Therefore, as the diagnosis of breast cancer is not specifically
listed as covered, we must deny coverage. However, GEHA now
participates in the National Cancer Institute sponsorship of a
clinical research trial involving the use of high dose
chemotherapy with autologous bone marrow transplant for the
treatment of breast cancer. Qualified applicants who undertake
the treatment at participating centers will be randomized into a
regimen of conventional treatment or treatment that uses high dose
chemotherapy with autologous bone marrow transplant. To obtain
more information, please call 800-225-0495. If you have any
questions, please advise.

Sincerely,

Richard B. Michelson, MD, MHSA
Medical Director

dkr

cc: Member
Ann Logan, RN

Congress of the United States
Washington, DC 20515

October 29, 1993

Honorable James King
Director
Office of Personnel Management
1900 E. Street, N.W.
Washington, DC 20415-0001

Dear Mr. King:

We are writing to request that you require Federal Employee
Health Benefits (FEHB) Program insurance carriers to cover
high-dose chemotherapy and autologous bone marrow
transplantation (HDC/ABMT) for breast cancer.

Insurance carriers such as Blue Cross/Blue Shield cover bone
marrow transplant treatment for testicular cancer, hodgkin's
disease, and other diseases but will not pay for breast
cancer. Yet, according to statistics from Duke University,
bone marrow transplant treatment for advanced breast cancer
is eight times more effective than conventional dose therapy.
Moreover, 72 percent of patients with high-risk cancer
involving ten or more lymph nodes are alive and disease-free
six years after HDC/ABMT. Only 30 to 35 percent of patients
who receive standard dose therapy are alive and disease-free
after six years.

One of our concerns is that breast cancer is being singled
out because it is widespread. There are 100,000 new breast
cancer cases each year. If even a small percentage of the
cases required treatment, it could cost millions of dollars.
But cost should not be the deciding factor.

We realize that there are clinical trials being conducted
with the National Cancer Institute. Unfortunately, the
trials seem to be a delaying tactic. They should have been
completed after two to three years but have been extended
another two years.

We urge you, based on extensive data that is already
available, to include bone marrow treatment for breast cancer
under existing plans.

Sincerely,

1.	Mike Parker (D-MS)	26.	Tom Lantos (D-CA)
2.	James A. Traficant Jr. (D-OH)	27.	John M. McHugh (R_NY)
3.	George Hochbrueckner (D-NY)	28.	Bob Filner (D-CA)
4.	Barney Frank (D-MA)	29.	Jerrold Nadler (D-NY)
5.	Senator Bennett Johnson (D-LA)	30.	John T. Myers (R-IN)
6.	Ileana Ros-Lehtinen (R-FL)	31.	W. G. Hefner (D-NC)
7.	Jay Inslee (D-WA)	32.	Stephen L. Neal (D-NC)
8.	Carrie Meek (D-FL)	33.	Pete King (R-NY)
9.	Ron Dellums (D-CA)	34.	Marcy Kaptur (D-OH)
10.	William Hughes (D-NJ)	35.	Patsy T. Mink (D-HI)
11.	Leslie Byrne (D-VA)	36.	Karen Thurmond (D-FL)
12.	Carlos Romero-Barcelo (D-PR)	37.	Bruce F. Vento (D-MN)
13.	Barbara Rose-Collins (D-MI)	38.	Martin Frost (D-TX)
14.	Joline Unsoeld (D-WA)	39.	Steny H. Hoyer (D-MD)
15.	Nancy Pelosi (D-CA)	40.	Anna Eshoo (D-CA)
16.	Lynn Woolsey (D-CA)	41.	Marilyn Lloyd (D-TN)
17.	Pete Stark (D-CA)	42.	Blanche Lambert (D-AR)
18.	Louise Slaughter (D-NY)	43.	Cynthia McKinney (D-GA)
19.	Maria Cantwell (D-WA)	44.	Dan Schaefer (R-CO)
20.	Senator Frank Lauttenberg (D-NJ)	45.	Frank McCloskey (D-IN)
21.	Corinne Brown (D-FL)	46.	Don Johnson (D-GA)
22.	Eleanor Holmes Norton (D DC)	47.	Thomas Foglietta (D-PA)
23.	Tom Sawyer (D-OH)	48.	Martin Frost (D-TX)
24.	John Conyers (D-MI)	49.	James Moran (D-VA)
25.	Gary Ackerman (D-NY)	50.	John Spratt (D-SC)
		51.	Senator Tom Harkin (D-IA)
		52.	Martin Meehan (D-MA)
		53.	Norman Mineta (D-CA)

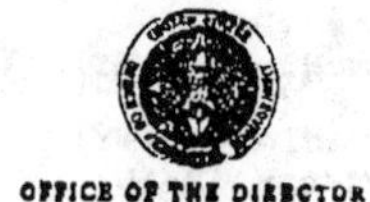

Honorable Eleanor Holmes Norton
U.S. House of Representatives
Washington, DC 20515

Dear Delegate Norton:

Thank you for your letter of October 29, 1993, concerning coverage for high-dose chemotherapy with autologous bone marrow transplantation (HDC/ABMT) for the treatment of breast cancer under the Federal Employees Health Benefits (FEHB) Program.

We too believe that FEHB carriers should cover treatments that have been demonstrated to be effective. Simply stated, the reason HDC/ABMT is covered for some treatments but not for breast cancer is that the treatment has not been shown to be more effective than conventional treatment for this particular disease. We know, however, that it carries a much higher degree of risk. Mandating coverage for such treatments is not a matter of cost; it's a matter of assuring that the treatments help more than they harm. This is precisely the question that the ongoing clinical trials are addressing.

The Duke University study referenced in your letter states that due to its toxicity, cost, and complexity, at present this treatment should only be offered at major centers of excellence in which patients are entered into randomized comparative trials whenever possible. The conclusion of the study is that evaluation in randomized clinical trials is warranted and currently underway. It does not recommend that HDC/ABMT for breast cancer be considered accepted medical practice or mainstreamed into conventional medicine. Based on this study, and other medical evidence that we have reviewed, we continue to believe that HDC/ABMT for the treatment of breast cancer is dangerous and its effectiveness unproven.

The National Cancer Institute (NCI) has also advised us that HDC/ABMT for breast cancer should not be performed outside the clinical trials setting. A number of FEHB plans, including the Government-wide Service Benefit Plan and several of the largest open fee-for-service plans, are participating in a demonstration project to offer Federal members the opportunity to participate in NCI-sponsored clinical trials studying HDC/ABMT for breast cancer in centers of excellence throughout the country. Duke University is a participant in this project as well.

Honorable Eleanor Holmes Norton   2

Through our participation in this demonstration project, the FEHB Program can
contribute to the effort to define the benefits of this treatment for patients with
breast cancer. As the Duke University study recommends, we are awaiting the
NCI trials results. We will not hesitate to modify our coverage requirements as
soon as reliable clinical evidence indicates that HDC/ABMT is at least as effective
as conventional treatment for breast cancer and is worth the added risk.

Thank you for the opportunity to respond to you on this issue of mutual concern.

Sincerely,

James B. King
Director